Rev. Dr. Christ(
Rev. Andy Cal(
Editors

Voices in Disability and Spirituality from the Land Down Under: Outback to Outfront

Voices in Disability and Spirituality from the Land Down Under: From Outback to Outfront has been co-published simultaneously as *Journal of Religion, Disability & Health*, Volume 8, Numbers 1/2 2004.

Pre-publication
REVIEWS,
COMMENTARIES,
EVALUATIONS . . .

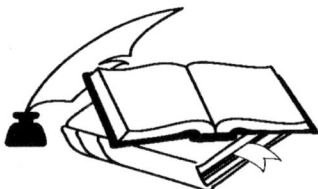

"In recent years disability theology has emerged alongside Black theology and women's theology as a new genre seeking to express the concerns of people whose experience has often been marginalized. This collection is A SIGNIFICANT AUSTRALIAN CONTRIBUTION TO THIS GROWING LITERATURE. The early explorers named Australia 'the south land of the Holy Spirit.' This collection reminds us that this is still a valid description of the sun-burnt country."

John M. Hull, PhD, Hon DTheol
Professor Emeritus of Religious Education
University of Birmingham, England
Author of On Sight and Insight
and In the Beginning There was Darkness

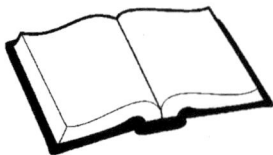

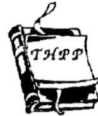

The Haworth Pastoral Press®
An Imprint of The Haworth Press, Inc.

New York • London • Victoria (AU)
www.HaworthPress.com

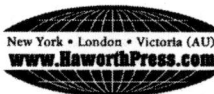

Voices in Disability and Spirituality from the Land Down Under: Outback to Outfront

Voices in Disability and Spirituality from the Land Down Under: Outback to Outfront has been co-published simultaneously as *Journal of Religion, Disability & Health*, Volume 8, Numbers 1/2 2004.

The *Journal of Religion, Disability & Health*™ Monographic "Separates"

(formerly the *Journal of Religion in Disability & Rehabilitation* series)*

Below is a list of "separates," which in serials librarianship means a special issue simultaneously published as a special journal issue or double-issue *and* as a "separate" hardbound monograph. (This is a format which we also call a "DocuSerial.")

"Separates" are published because specialized libraries or professionals may wish to purchase a specific thematic issue by itself in a format which can be separately cataloged and shelved, as opposed to purchas-ing the journal on an on-going basis. Faculty members may also more easily consider a "separate" for classroom adoption.

"Separates" are carefully classified separately with the major book jobbers so that the journal tie-in can be noted on new book order slips to avoid duplicate purchasing.

You may wish to visit Haworth's website at . . .

http://www.HaworthPress.com

. . . to search our online catalog for complete tables of contents of these separates and related publications.

You may also call 1-800-HAWORTH (outside US/Canada: 607-722-5857), or Fax 1-800-895-0582 (out-side US/Canada: 607-771-0012), or e-mail at:

docdelivery@haworthpress.com

Voices in Disability and Spirituality from the Land Down Under: From Outback to Outfront, edited by Rev. Dr. Christopher Newell, PhD, and Rev. Andy Calder (Vol. 8, No. 1/2, 2004). *"In recent years disability theology has emerged alongside Black theology and womens' theology as a new genre seeking to express the concerns of people whose experience has often been marginalized. This collection is A SIGNIFICANT AUSTRALIAN CONTRIBUTION TO THIS GROWING LITERATURE. The early explorers named Australia 'the south land of the Holy Spirit.' John M. Hull, PhD, Hon DTheol, Professor Emeritus of Religious Education, University of Birmingham, England; Author of* On Sight and Insight *and* In the Beginning There was Dark-ness).

Graduate Theological Education and the Human Experience of Disability, edited by Robert C. Anderson (Vol. 7, No. 3, 2003). *"A comprehensive overview of theological education and disability. . . . Concise and well written. . . . Offers rich theological insights and abundant practical advice. I strongly recommend this volume as a key introduction to this important emerging topic in theological education." (Rev. John W. Crossin, PhD, OSFS, Executive Director, Washington Theological Consortium)*

The Pastoral Voice of Robert Perske, edited by William C. Gaventa, Jr., MDiv, and David L. Coulter, MD (Vol. 7, No. 1/2, 2003). *"Must reading for seminary students and clinincal program directors. Pastors, providers, and parents concerned with persons suffering from cognitive, intellectual, and developmental disabilities will find these vigorous testimonies readable, timely, fresh, and inspiring despite having been written more than 30 years ago." (Barbara J. Lampe, JD, Executive Director, National Apostolate for Inclusion Ministry)*

Spirituality and Intellectual Disability: International Perspectives on the Effect of Culture and Religion on Healing Body, Mind, and Soul, edited by William C. Gaventa, Jr., MDiv, and David L. Coulter, MD (Vol. 5, No. 2/3, 2001). *"Must reading . . . perspectives from many faiths and cultures on the spiritual needs and gifts of people with mental retardation." (Ginny Thornburgh, EdM, Religion and Disability Program, National Organization on Disability, Washington, DC)*

The Theological Voice of Wolf Wolfensberger, edited by William C. Gaventa, MDiv, and David L. Coulter, MD (Vol. 4, No. 2/3, 2001). *This thought-provoking volume presents Wolfensberger's challenging, outrageous, and inspiring ideas on the theological significance of disabilities, including the problem with wheelchair access ramps in churches, the meaning of suffering, and the spiritual gifts of the mentally retarded.*

A Look Back: The Birth of the Americans With Disabilities Act, edited by Robert C. Anderson, MDiv (Vol. 2, No. 4, 1996).* *Takes you to the unique moment in American history when persons* *of many different backgrounds and with different disabilities united to press Congress for full recognition and protection of their rights as American citizens.*

Pastoral Care of the Mentally Disabled: Advancing Care of the Whole Person, edited by Sally K. Severino, MD, and Reverend Richard Liew, PhD (Vol. 1, No. 2, 1994).* *"A great book for theologians with a refreshing dogma-free approach; thought provoking for physiotherapists and all other human beings!" (The Chartered Society of Physiotherapy)*

Voices in Disability and Spirituality from the Land Down Under: Outback to Outfront

Rev. Dr. Christopher Newell
Rev. Andy Calder
Editors

Voices in Disability and Spirituality from the Land Down Under: Outback to Outfront has been co-published simultaneously as *Journal of Religion, Disability & Health*, Volume 8, Numbers 1/2 2004.

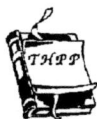

The Haworth Pastoral Press®
An Imprint of The Haworth Press, Inc.

New York • London • Victoria (AU)
www.HaworthPress.com

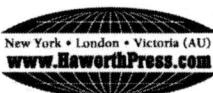

Published by

The Haworth Pastoral Press, 10 Alice Street, Binghamton, NY 13904-1580 USA

The Haworth Pastoral Press is an imprint of The Haworth Press, Inc., 10 Alice Street, Binghamton, NY 13904-1580 USA.

Voices in Disability and Spirituality from the Land Down Under: Outback to Outfront has been co-published simultaneously as *Journal of Religion, Disability & Health*, Volume 8, Numbers 1/2 2004.

The development, preparation, and publication of this work has been undertaken with great care. However, the publisher, employees, editors, and agents of The Haworth Press and all imprints of The Haworth Press, Inc., including The Haworth Medical Press® and The Pharmaceutical Products Press®, are not responsible for any errors contained herein or for consequences that may ensue from use of materials or information contained in this work. Opinions expressed by the author(s) are not necessarily those of The Haworth Press, Inc.

Cover design by Jennifer Gaska

Front cover photographs by B.P. Calder. Printed with permission.
Top photo: Yellow Waters, Northern Territory, Australia
Bottom photo: Uluru, Northern Territory, Australia

Library of Congress Cataloging-in-Publication Data

Voices in disability and spirituality from the Land Down Under: outback to outfront / Christopher Newell, Andy Calder, editors.
     p. cm.
    "Co-published simultaneously as Journal of religion, disability & health, volume 8, numbers 1/2 2004"–T.p. verso.
    Includes bibliographical references and index.
    ISBN 0-7890-2607-4 (hard cover : alk. paper)–ISBN 0-7890-2608-2 (soft cover : alk. paper)
    1. People with disabilities–Religious life–Australia–Congresses I. Newell, Christopher, 1964- II. Calder, Andy.
BL625.9.P45V65 2004
201'.7624'0994–dc22   2004009975

Indexing, Abstracting & Website/Internet Coverage

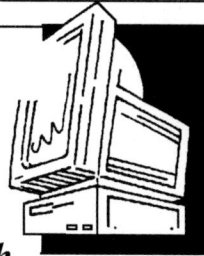

Journal of Religion, Disability & Health

This section provides you with a list of major indexing & abstracting services. That is to say, each service began covering this periodical during the year noted in the right column. Most Websites which are listed below have indicated that they will either post, disseminate, compile, archive, cite or alert their own Website users with research-based content from this work. (This list is as current as the copyright date of this publication.)

Abstracting, Website/Indexing Coverage . . . . Year When Coverage Began

- *Applied Social Sciences Index & Abstracts (ASSIA)*
  (Online: ASSI via Data-Star) (CDRom: ASSIA Plus)
  <http://www.csa.com> 1994
- *AURSI African Urban & Regional Science Index. A scholarly &*
  research index which synthesises & compiles all publications
  on urbanization & regional science in Africa within the world.
  Published annually 2004
- *CINAHL (Cumulative Index to Nursing & Allied Health*
  Literature), in print, EBSCO, and SilverPlatter, Data-Star,
  and PaperChase (Support materials include Subject Heading List,
  Database Search Guide, and instructional video)
  <http://www.cinahl.com> 1994
- *Educational Research Abstracts (ERA) (online database)*
  <http://www.tandf.co.uk/era> 2003
- *e-psyche, LLC <http://www.e-psyche.net>* 2002
- *Family & Society Studies Worldwide*
  <http://www.nisc.com> 1996
- *Family Index Database*
  <http://www.familyscholar.com> 2003
- *Human Resources Abstracts (HRA)* 1994

- *IBZ International Bibliography of Periodical Literature*
  <http://www.saur.de> International Bibliographie
  der geistes- und socialwissenschaftlichen Zeitschriftenliteratur
  See IBZ 1996

(continued)

Special Bibliographic Notes related to special journal issues (separates) and indexing/abstracting:

- indexing/abstracting services in this list will also cover material in any "separate" that is co-published simultaneously with Haworth's special thematic journal issue or DocuSerial. Indexing/abstracting usually covers material at the article/chapter level.
- monographic co-editions are intended for either non-subscribers or libraries which intend to purchase a second copy for their circulating collections.
- monographic co-editions are reported to all jobbers/wholesalers/approval plans. The source journal is listed as the "series" to assist the prevention of duplicate purchasing in the same manner utilized for books-in-series.
- to facilitate user/access services all indexing/abstracting services are encouraged to utilize the co-indexing entry note indicated at the bottom of the first page of each article/chapter/contribution.
- this is intended to assist a library user of any reference tool (whether print, electronic, online, or CD-ROM) to locate the monographic version if the library has purchased this version but not a subscription to the source journal.
- individual articles/chapters in any Haworth publication are also available through the Haworth Document Delivery Service (HDDS).

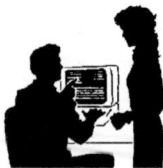

Voices in Disability and Spirituality from the Land Down Under: Outback to Outfront

CONTENTS

ABOUT THE EDITORS

The Reverend Dr. Christopher Newell is Associate Professor of Medical Ethics in the University of Tasmania's School of Medicine. He also supervises doctoral research for LaTrobe University (Victoria) and the Melbourne College of Divinity. As a consultant, Dr. Newell has an ongoing involvement with the provision of advice to corporations and Australian Government bodies, universities, and community sector organizations. From 1994-2000 he was Vice President of the Australian Bioethics Association. He is also an Angelican priest, currently on staff at St. David's Cathedral in Hobart, and a member of the Tasmanian Government's Disability Policy Steering Committee, appointed by the Tasmanian Premier. In addition, he chairs the Disability Advisory Board of the Australian Communications Industry Forum, and is a member of the boards of the Consumers' Health Forum of Australia and the Disability Studies and Research Institute.

Reverend Andy Calder is Senior Chaplain at the Epworth Hospital, Australia's largest not-for-profit hospital. He served previously as a chaplain with Prahran Mission, a support service for people experiencing mental illness, and as Coordinator of Disability Services for the synod of Victoria Uniting Church in Australia. In this role, Reverend Calder encouraged the inclusion of people with disabilities into all aspects of church life. A major component was the development of the Disability Action Plan, which was endorsed by the Australian Human Rights and Equal Opportunity Commission. Reverend Calder is a member of the Human Research and Ethics Committees of the Epworth Hospital and Scope (formerly the Spastic Society), and was the convenor of the third Australian Disability and Spirituality Conference, which provided the impetus for the writing of this book.

Foreword

From many parts of the world, and especially North America and Europe, Australia is a long ways away. For many, the immediate images and metaphors are sometimes ones with negative implications we also associate with the world(s) of disability: far away, down under, strange, different, scary, big, desert, dangerous. When I first went to Australia in 1998, I also learned that many Aussies have a kind of inferiority complex, sometimes from those negative implications, but also from Americans and others whom they have perceived as always coming to Australia to tell or show them how things really should be done.

If it does anything, this volume should dispel a few of those stereotypes, images, and assumptions, for this collection of writings and perspectives is a huge gift to the rest of the world and to the worldwide field of disability and spirituality. To reverse an Australian metaphor, these poppies stand tall, and should be proud to do so. One reason for that claim is its genesis in the Third (yes, *third*) National Conference on Spirituality and Disability in Australia, Exclusion and Embrace, held in October of 2001 in Melbourne. How many other countries have had that many interfaith and interdisciplinary national conferences focusing on this area of ministry, service, and reflection? Another has been held since then in New Zealand, with another being planned for the latter part of 2004 in Sydney. That rich recent history is built on some long time work as you will see in some of the article by Drs. Steer and Gale about the religious origins of many disability services in Australia and current, comprehensive work done by the Uniting Church in Australia (Wansbrough and Cooper) and other faith groups, such as the Roman Catholic Archdiocese of

[Haworth co-indexing entry note]: "Foreword." Gaventa, Bill. Co-published simultaneously in *Journal of Religion, Disability & Health* (The Haworth Pastoral Press, an imprint of The Haworth Press, Inc.) Vol. 8, No. 1/2, 2004, pp. xvii-xx; and: *Voices in Disability and Spirituality from the Land Down Under: Outback to Outfront* (eds: Rev. Dr. Christopher Newell and Rev. Andy Calder) The Haworth Pastoral Press, an imprint of The Haworth Press, Inc., 2004, pp. xiii-xvi. Single or multiple copies of this article are available for a fee from The Haworth Document Delivery Service [1-800-HAWORTH, 9:00 a.m. - 5:00 p.m. (EST). E-mail address: docdelivery@haworthpress.com].

xiii

Brisbane. I would also include a booklet written by South Australian Dr. Norm Habel in the International Year of the Disabled in 1980, *Is Christ Disabled?*, a wonderful series of four Biblical reflections for use in congregations which I have illegally smuggled into congregations for years.

But it is not just the history. This volume is also a metaphor of the way that images and experience from a "foreign" land, like the lands or worlds of disability, can become images and metaphors that speak to everyone, empowering all of us to look in our own unique environments and experiences to find treasures that enrich us all.

Christopher Newell and Andy Calder start it off with their Introduction that transforms the image of desert in ways that are similar to Kathleen Norris's great quote in her book about the bleak landscape of North Dakota in the U.S., *Dakota: A Spiritual Geography*, "The places one assumes to be empty are full of the angels of God. (Norris, 1993). Andy Calder continues that movement with the metaphor of the Australian verandah, that place around the house between the inside and outside, the home and the big world, where conversation can and needs to happen that bridges both worlds. The Australian clichés he analyzes have their own versions in many places of the world. The unique perspective is to look at them, and the Biblical/theological foundations, from the perspective of that verandah. Jayne Clapton brings the image of the explorer/conqueror from the Australian past to the strange new world of genetics and bioethics, using it to pose the wonderful question of whether those who profess to help in the world of disabilities are adventurers and aids, or scientific (or religious) imperialists who come to colonize and control. Lorna Hallahan speaks from the Australian experience of those who have immigrated there (either voluntarily or, as at first, involuntarily, in the shipment of convicts) in the search for community: community is not a destination, but a moral journey, defined by those who reach across the gaps in relationships with others.

Then we have two voices in Peter Hawkins and Melinda Jones that represent some of what is the rich religious and cultural diversity that is Australia. One is the first article that I can remember in the *Journal of Religion, Disability & Health's* history that explores a current relationship with the world of disability from a Buddhist perspective, other than the volume of M. Miles [6 (2/3)] writings that explores Eastern cultural attitudes and historical writings. (Please note that since the time this article was written, Peter W. Hawkins has become a Buddhist monk, now known as Thich Truc Thong Phap.) The next article is by an Orthodox Jew, a mother, and a lawyer, with one of the best overall summaries of Jewish perspectives about disability that I can remember, period. Both do a wonderful job of noting the difference between what a faith tradition teaches, and the actual current practice. Both then draw upon the tradition to inspire and infuse current practice, and cite examples that illustrate the heart of their respective traditions at their best.

Melinda Jones notes that Jewish spirituality imbues the material world with meaning, and thus seeks the divine in the ordinary and everyday. Sometimes Christians and other faiths think that is too "secular." When and if you go to Australia, you may hear, as I often did, a sense of apology for what many there think is the thoroughly "secular" nature of their society. One could illustrate that with one of my favorite ads which I saw while there: a picture of the MCG (Melbourne Cricket Grounds . . . the biggest stadium), full, on a Sunday, for cricket or Aussie football game, with the inscription, *"Come and Visit our Place of Worship."*

But that assessment is far too shallow, in my opinion and experience. For one, the original inhabitants of Australia, the Aborigines, have known for centuries that it is a land imbued and infused with an amazing sense of spirit and spirituality. Unfortunately, we don't have an aboriginal voice in this collection, but there are several articles which explore that question about whether the "secular" is separate from the "sacred." Christopher Newell and Pam McGrath describe a powerful case story about the sacredness of human connection and support. Leonie Reid describes the mutuality of giving and receiving in personal advocacy services with people with disabilities in far West Australia. Lyn Dowling looks at the ways that efforts to help staff and students in a "secular" school for children with disabilities deal with grief, death, and loss leads to new rituals and ways of honoring spiritual feelings, experience, and depths. Finally, Elizabeth Mosely, in her poetic voice, describes her experience when that which is supposedly "sacred" turns out to be a rejecting place for a person with a disability who seeks to live out his or her spirituality and faith. Her question about a new cathedral is "Does the building welcome?", reminding us that a hostile environment to either spirituality or disability can occur in both "secular" and "sacred" places.

As readers of the Journal already know, my trip to Australia for the Melbourne conference which gave birth to this collection led to a moment that was perhaps the most sacred moment in my life (Grace Down Under)[2]. So I partly feel like a returning adventurer, profoundly grateful for the slavish toil of Christopher Newell and Andy Calder as collectors and editors of this edition, and the hard work of all of its authors. But I remember a popular postcard in Australia that captures the same sense of reversal of perspective that we often feel in the world of spirituality and disability. In this postcard, Australia is in the Northern Hemisphere, in the center of the map, and North America, Europe, and Asian in the Southern. Thus our title: *Voices in Disability and Spirituality from the Land Down Under: Outback to Outfront.*

I hope and trust you as readers will learn as much from them as I have, and that we will also learn how to see our worlds, environments, and relationships with new images of adventure, mystery, holiness, and revelation. May we all learn the Australian blessing for that kind of hard work and endeavor that gifts us all: "Good on yer, mates."

Bill Gaventa
Co-Editor
Journal of Religion, Disability & Health

REFERENCES

Gaventa, W. (2002). Grace Down Under. *Journal of Religion, Disability & Health.* 6(1). Binghamton: The Haworth Press, Inc., pp. 89-95.

Miles, M. (Ed). (2002). Disability in Asian Cultures and Beliefs: History and Service Development. *Journal of Religion, Disability & Health* 6(2/3). Binghamton: The Haworth Press, Inc.

Norris, Kathleen (1993) *Dakota: A Spiritual Geography.* New York: Houghton-Mifflin Company.

Introduction:
An Antipodean Perspective
on Disability and Spirituality

Christopher Newell, MDiv
Andy Calder, BBSc, BTheol, DipRec

What should a special Australian collection look like? If we are to believe the stereotypes, then it may well be that the bronzed body should figure prominently, or the theme of sand and surf, or, indeed, the experience of desert. If we think about the Australian icons which featured prominently in the opening ceremony of the 2000 Olympics, then to those images we can add the non-disabled lifesaver with zinc appropriately smeared on the nose, or even the famous Hills hoist clothesline. A famous Australian invention and cultural icon, the Hills hoist points to our highly urbanised culture and important dream of owning a house with a backyard. Of course, when we look a little deeper, we need to move beyond the stereotypes of Australia, since over 85% of the population lives in urban locations.

At first glance, some of the articles in this issue do not explore disability in terms of religiousness. Yet, when we look a little closer we can actually discover that all of these articles are testimony to the nature of contemporary Australian spirituality commented upon by David Tacey in a variety of books including his latest contribution, *The Spirituality Revolution*. As Tacey writes:

[Haworth co-indexing entry note]: "Introduction: An Antipodean Perspective on Disability and Spirituality." Newell, Christopher, and Andy Calder. Co-published simultaneously in *Journal of Religion, Disability & Health* (The Haworth Pastoral Press, an imprint of The Haworth Press, Inc.) Vol. 8, No. 1/2, 2004, pp. 1-3; and: *Voices in Disability and Spirituality from the Land Down Under: Outback to Outfront* (ed: Christopher Newell, and Andy Calder) The Haworth Pastoral Press, an imprint of The Haworth Press, Inc., 2004, pp. 1-3. Single or multiple copies of this article are available for a fee from The Haworth Document Delivery Service [1-800-HAWORTH, 9:00 a.m. - 5:00 p.m. (EST). E-mail address: docdelivery@haworthpress.com].

Whatever its cause, social alienation is a reality and keenly experienced today. To fall out of society and into the dark unknown can be extremely disorienting and unpleasant. . . . But the fall out of social identification can also be a *felix culpa*, a fortunate fall, if the individual is able to find his or her way to the underground stream that brings renewal and healing. The way is precarious and the path is dark and uncertain, but an encounter with the spirit brings new vitality. Paradoxically, the spirit thrusts the wandering soul back into life and returns him or her to the surface, with renewed enthusiasm and commitment for the work that has to be done. True spirit will not drag down and destroy, because its passion is to revitalise life and transform the ordinary world by its extraordinary power. Thus, the fortunate fall can lead to reversals, conversions and prophetic commitment to a new sense of destiny or purpose. Down and out one minute, the individual can suddenly find him or her self hurled back into life and serving a greater will with considerable verve and gusto.[1]

When we take as the starting point of our analysis the quest for meaning and the spirituality of people, then these papers reflect some deep strains of spirituality and an emerging dimension of Australian spirituality with regard to disability. As some of the articles in the collection and the Australian conferences on disability and spirituality which have occurred in Brisbane (1996), Adelaide (1998) and Melbourne (2001) attest, many Australians with disabilities have been hurt by religious attitudes which are uncritically informed by dominant understandings of disability in terms of deficit and charity. Some of these papers document a key dimension of Australia–the desert–the spiritual desert which many of us have experienced. Yet, when we look a little deeper, we find that the desert, and indeed the experience of Australians with disabilities and those who care for them, actually is not devoid of life; it is a desert teeming with life. That is, it could be, if only we have the courage and perspective to realise this.

In Australia there are some good programs funded by faith communities, with regard to the embrace of people with disabilities. Yet the fact that such special programs need to exist at all highlights significant problems existent in established faith communities (as people and structures) as they routinely create people with disabilities as *other*.

We would suggest that it is only when the Australian congregations and faith communities routinely and purposefully embrace people with disabilities in direct relationship that some of the significant problems will start to be dealt with systematically. In Christian terms, this requires significant *doing* of theology: re-thinking who belongs to the household of God and who is routinely consigned to the desert or to the crashing waves of the surf.

The 2000 Sydney Olympics was remarkable for its portrayal of Australian icons and stereotypical images which failed to depict disability. The one cameo performance at the opening ceremony was that of Betty Cuthbert, a former Olympian who appeared momentarily in her wheelchair before the whole non-disabled Olympic experience moved on, comfortable that people with disabilities would be attended to in a separate Paralympics. Perhaps it is only when disability is routinely and thoroughly celebrated as an integral part of Australian iconism and imagery that we will see an Australian spirituality, and religious institutions, which truly embrace people with disabilities.

Our thanks to the various people who made this special volume possible; especially the anonymous referees and to Alex Fitzpatrick for her role as sub-editor.

NOTE

1. Tacey, D. *The Spirituality Revolution*, Harper Collins, Sydney, 2003, p. 54.

"God Has Chosen This for You"– "Really?" A Pastoral and Theological Appraisal of This and Some Other Well-Known Clichés Used in Australia to Support People with Disabilities

Reverend Andy Calder, BBSc, BTheol, DipRec

SUMMARY. The author explores and critiques some Australian quotations often used to purportedly comfort and support people with disabilities, their families and carers. It is contended that these "God is on your side" clichés are, at best, problematic, and, at worst, instill spiritual trauma upon the recipient, as they perpetuate a sense of victimhood and collusion by God in their suffering. In exploring some of the theology and Christian healing narratives which lie behind these clichés, alternative pastoral responses are proposed; such as companionship, nurture and listening within networks of support and friendship. The Australian verandah is used as a metaphor for the 'in-between place' where a range

Reverend Andy Calder was Disability Resources Minister, Uniting Church in Australia, Synod of Victoria when he wrote this article. He is currently Senior Chaplain, Epworth Hospital, Richmond, Victoria and a Clinical Pastoral Education Supervisor.

Address correspondence to: Rev. Andy Calder, 141 Ramsden Street, Clifton Hill, Victoria, Australia, 3068 (E-mail: andyc@epworth.org.au).

[Haworth co-indexing entry note]: "God Has Chosen This for You"–"Really?" A Pastoral and Theological Appraisal of This and Some Other Well-Known Clichés Used in Australia to Support People with Disabilities." Calder, Reverend Andy. Co-published simultaneously in *Journal of Religion, Disability & Health* (The Haworth Pastoral Press, an imprint of The Haworth Press, Inc.) Vol. 8, No. 1/2, 2004, pp. 5-19; and: *Voices in Disability and Spirituality from the Land Down Under: Outback to Outfront* (ed: Christopher Newell, and Andy Calder) The Haworth Pastoral Press, an imprint of The Haworth Press, Inc., 2004, pp. 5-19. Single or multiple copies of this article are available for a fee from The Haworth Document Delivery Service [1-800-HAWORTH, 9:00 a.m. - 5:00 p.m. (EST). E-mail address: docdelivery@haworthpress.com].

http://www.haworthpress.com/web/JRDH
Digital Object Identifier: 10.1300/J095v8n01_02

of vistas and perspectives, looking both within and beyond, may help to illuminate an appropriate pastoral response. *[Article copies available for a fee from The Haworth Document Delivery Service: 1-800-HAWORTH. E-mail address: <docdelivery@haworthpress.com> Website: <http://www.HaworthPress.com> © 2004 by The Haworth Press, Inc. All rights reserved.]*

KEYWORDS. Disability, theology, pastoral care

During the 1980s I worked with the respite holiday camping program at Noahs Ark Toy Library, a community-based service in Melbourne, Victoria, for children with disabilities and their families. I became aware of certain clichés that the parents of these children were sometimes offered in order to console or support them. Fullwood and Cronin name them the "God is on your side" clichés (1986, pp. 90-93). They include clichés like *God has blessed you with this gift–you are a lucky couple*; *God has chosen this for you*; *It's a test of your faith*; *These things are meant to be*; *We all have our crosses to carry*. At the time, I uncritically accepted that such sayings were indeed of comfort and support to people trying to make sense of their altered family experience. I no longer believe this to be the case.

Ongoing involvement with people who live with disability, personal experience of disability through road trauma, and some theological study have led me to revisit such clichés to determine their appropriateness, or otherwise, as pastoral responses. I contend that such clichés are, at best, problematic and, at worst, very damaging, and result in spiritual abuse and trauma. Recipients say that these clichés lead to increased feelings of guilt, blame and shame, a sense of passivity, and confusion about the divine intent–*is God for or against me?* In this article, I am hoping to explore further my own theology of disability, and propose some pastoral responses which counter these clichés.

What gives rise to these clichés? Presumably, they are inherited from family and other influences within society and culture. They are carried subconsciously and are expressed when a particular circumstance of disability is confronted. Deeper than that, they are an abiding expression of a cause-and-effect dynamic in which God is being pronounced as one who has somehow willed this circumstance upon these people who, for whatever reason, have been chosen as the bearers of God's displeasure. People hear them as clichés of judgement–of God being against them. The recipients are cast as people whose faith is perhaps suspect, as people who have perhaps incurred God's wrath for some misdeed, and as people who have no control over their circumstances: indeed, as victims.

Many people experience disability as giving rise to a heightened sense of shame and exclusion–*shame* in the sense of being disrespected or considered deviant or different because of stereotyped images of what is supposedly 'normal.' People are stared at or viewed as a 'problem' to be 'fixed,' rather than as a person in their own right with all the richness, diversity and paradox of our human existence. Shame here is not being correlated with guilt or having done something wrong; rather, with a sense of negative self-worth, of rejection, of other people's awkwardness, of being dishonored and of being patronized. The God-is-on-your-side clichés are a distancing device. How does one reply to such prescriptive and categorical assertions in the midst of shame, grief or trauma, especially when God is invoked in such definitive terms?

It is my contention that individuals with disabilities, parents, siblings and extended families who are the recipients of such clichés are at risk of becoming further alienated from the very faith tradition which is called to be an agent of reconciliation in the name of Christ. In the exploration of these questions, this article will draw on a range of literature, illustrative of personal experience and interpretation, in addition to writers who explore the impact of traditional understandings of the biblical healing stories.

Australia is a vast land–the largest island continent in the world. Its 20 million people are predominantly coastal dwellers. At its geographic heart is Uluru, the desert site sacred to Indigenous Australians, known more widely to an international audience as Ayers Rock. This sacred place is increasingly being visited by Australians. There are differing views about the Australian psyche in relation to desert and coast. Tacey (1995) identifies the center as being the location of our spiritual identity; a place of metaphorical and literal journey to the desert or inner place where transformation occurs. Pickard (1998) offers another perspective: being people who live at the intersection of land, sea and sky, we are a people looking both outwards and inwards. He points out the need for theological conversations to inhabit a place that is neither on the inside nor the outside but in-between, and for this he utilizes the image of a verandah. We are a verandah people, and God is to be found in the "in-between places" of our existence. It is noteworthy that the verandah is an icon of particular importance in defining Australian dwellings and shelter from a hostile environment. This article will draw on Pickard's metaphor of the verandah to explore a response that takes account of both internal and external vistas.

A major issue for some people with disabilities is how the Christian tradition offers and interprets the meaning of the healing stories in the scriptures. Is it healing or cure that people are seeking? Is it healing or cure that the tradition offers, and is this necessarily physical? Returning to the cause-and-effect dynamic implicit in the God-is-on-your-side clichés, I wish to explore the issue of healing by looking at the following four aspects: (i) faith or faithlessness;

(ii) disability as a reflection of evil; (iii) the relationship of sin and disability; and (iv) suffering being a sign of God's will. This exploration will take place within the ambiguity of two New Testament healing stories: the story of the paralyzed man (in Mark chapter 2), and the man born blind (in John chapter 9). Arising from this, will be the proposition of pastoral responses that offer alternatives to the God-is-on-your-side clichés.

The distinction between healing and cure is well made by Senior (1995), writing about religion and disability:

> I use the term *cure* in a strict physical sense, referring to physical transformation by which, for example, the withered arm of the man in the synagogue of Capernaum is made straight. *Healing* has a more profound and comprehensive meaning, referring not only to physical transformation but to a profound spiritual transformation as well. Not all people–even in the drama of the gospels–have access to a cure; but all are invited to be healed. Even Jesus himself, one could say, would ultimately not experience cure but would be healed through the experience of resurrection. (pp. 12-13)

There are countless stories of people with disabilities who have sought a cure in vain, and have been left seriously doubting their faith. It is true that there are also some accounts of people being mysteriously and miraculously cured who have ascribed this to a faithful pursuit of healing, and these stories are not to be discounted. However, overwhelmingly, people have been driven to seek a cure because of a dominant and disabling theology that equates disabilities with sin. From codes of purity to acts of Jesus' healing, the implicit theological assumptions are that perfect bodies are equated with wholeness of spirit. Furthermore, Chopp (in Eiesland, 1994) suggests that:

> . . . as if to ensure the quest for purity, physical afflictions become elevated to virtuous suffering when, and only when, they can be spoken of as trials of obedience. Such teachings allow either one of two options for those with disabilities: miraculous healing or heroic suffering. (p. 11)

Is the emphasis on either of these options acceptable or helpful for people with disabilities grappling with everyday life? I believe not. The active pursuit of unfulfilled miraculous healing has left many a person with feelings of guilt and failure, whilst heroic suffering is likely to cast people as victims with diminished personal control and person-hood. The God-is-on-your-side clichés certainly reflect this passive notion of heroic suffering.

These two options of miraculous healing and heroic suffering reinforce theology and beliefs which emphasize the pursuit of 'ableness' and perfection.

This is astonishing when it is considered that Christian theology does not have an able-bodied God as its primal image. Rather, God offers grace through a broken body, and this is at the center of prayer, worship and mission. Eiesland (1994) has completed some groundbreaking work in developing a theology of liberation for people with disabilities, expounding upon the theology of a "Disabled God" in whom:

> ... the resurrection, the transcendence and perfection of God reveals true person-hood in the ordinariness of life. In this central symbol, full person-hood is not presented by the negation, belittlement, or repression of persons with disabilities. The Disabled God represents full person-hood as fully compatible with the experience of disability. (p. 11)

The story in chapter 2 of Mark's Gospel, of the paralyzed man who is lowered down through the roof illustrates the common belief in the first century of divine retribution, i.e., that a person's suffering is proportionate to his or her sin. Thus this story also reflects the implicit cause-and-effect contained within the God-is-on-your-side clichés. The theological progression of this cause-and-effect worldview is that any suffering on account of impairment or affliction is the result of some prior sin or evil. It also follows, as can be read in Psalm 32 for example, that any healing is seen as a sign of God's forgiveness of sin.

Furthermore, in this story of the paralyzed man, Jesus reflects the same basic worldview which links sin with disability. Jesus also emphasizes the faith of the four stretcher-bearers as being integral to the restoration of the man's mobility, and raises the ire of the Pharisees by proclaiming forgiveness of the man's sins. All the elements of the story reinforce the age-old notion that blemish and 'imperfection' are the result of sin. Within most biblical healing stories, the expressed presence of faith, be it in the person seeking healing, or in that of others, is central to the outcome of the encounter with Jesus.

And so, how might people react when told that their personal situation is a 'test of their faith?' Lane, quoted by Eiesland, writes with concern about the implication that those who are not healed must not have enough faith:

> Healing is expected to change the person who has a disability into one who does not. The burden of healing is placed totally on the person who is disabled, causing further suffering and continued alienation from the Church. (Lane, cited in Eiesland, 1994, p. 117)

A recurring theme of the healing stories is the restoration to full communal life. Indeed, one can well imagine the joy of the paralyzed man, once he got over the initial shock, of learning to walk again and taking part in all the things that previously he could only have dreamed about. This story and other healing stories are representative of inclusion in God's reign, but they raise the hermeneutic problem of why physical restoration is suggested as a precondition of entry into the community of faith. Why do people need to be seen as cured, in order to be accepted? Tiffany and Ringe (1996) raise the alarm bells of ecclesial hegemony when they raise questions such as:

> Why is such a premium placed on able-bodiedness? Why is the "good news" not expressed as a world made accessible to and accepting of persons of all physical, mental and psychological circumstances, rather than as persons changed to conform to the world's norms? (p. 183)

The emphasis here is on a radical shift from changing the 'form' of the individual to changing the 'form' of the environment which so often excludes and patronizes people who are seen as 'not fitting the mould.' A shift has gained impetus over recent decades in which the dominant biomedical conceptualization of disability has needed to increasingly recognize the social model of disability, and in which people with disabilities have asserted their rights of citizenship and equal participation.

Fulcher notes this shift in her discourse about the historical spectrum of meaning associated with disability (1989, pp. 21-41). She asserts that disability is a political and social construct which has been used to regulate people with disabilities. Whilst the practice of pastoral care has historically been shaped by and linked to the medical, lay and charity discourses, with their clinical concern for the body and its treatment, Fulcher's other two discourses on disability, rights and corporate, suggest that pastoral care be open to and mindful of its activity in the wider social discourse–how might it influence the form of the environment which so often alienates people? The sins of stereotyping and exclusion are trumpeted by many advocates and are enshrined in legislation to minimize their impact. This is a major contribution to healing and restoration of full communal life, which the church, looking out from the verandah, is also called to be part of.

With respect to the healing accounts and the sin-disability nexus, Grant (1998) asserts that there is no easy reconciliation between the healing stories and a vision of full and open participation of people with disabilities in the life of the church. However, she believes that the story of the man who was born blind, in Chapter 9 of John's gospel, offers an alternative perspective to some of the hermeneutic difficulties mentioned previously. There are three aspects, in particular, of Grant's writings which are pertinent to the considerations of this essay and which inform the alternative pastoral response to the God-is-on-your-side clichés.

Firstly, in responding to the disciples' question, "Rabbi, who sinned, this man or his parents that he was born blind?" (John 9:2), Jesus goes on to refute their assumptions of sin necessarily being the cause. In overturning the so-called traditional Jewish view of disability, it is tempting to appropriate this position and apply it universally. However, Grant points out that great caution should always be exercised before portraying Jesus as one who overturns 'backward' Jewish thinking. She refers to the writings of Bultmann on this text, when he says:

> . . . what Jesus says does not confute the Jewish position nor does it suggest that there is another way of looking at such cases . . . the saying is only concerned with the particular case in question at the moment. (Bultmann cited in Grant, 1998, p. 80)

However, it does open the door for a revised understanding and conversation about the intent of Jesus and the notion of the cause-and-effect formula of disability as the direct result of individual sin. In the light of contemporary understandings of genetic and environmental influences, the nuances of a particular circumstance give rise to a far more complex conclusion, if in fact a definitive one can be reached at all.

Secondly, according to Grant, it is interesting that the blind man has not asked for healing, nor does Jesus ask about the man's faith. The healing takes place unconditionally, without any stated expectations on the part of either the one healed or the healer. When the man returns from the Pool of Siloam, what develops throughout the interrogatory dialogue is the clarity of the man's identity in relation to his religious teachers, his family and neighbors, and Jesus who has healed him. For those who knew him, 'blindness' was his defining characteristic. But this man, with his bold and courageous rejoinders, asserts that his disability was never his defining characteristic. He knows himself to be the same person, blind or sighted, who wishes to respond to the call of discipleship and faith by demonstrating that God is at work in his life. Jesus did the work of faith and healing when he replied that no-one sinned; thus lifting one of the many burdens projected onto people with disabilities.

This third aspect of Grant's interpretation, along with the second observation that Jesus did not inquire about the depth of the man's faith, provide hopeful alternative messages to people wondering if they are faithful enough. They, in turn, can know that they are loved and accepted unconditionally by God, regardless of others' perceptions and prejudices or stigmatization. Alternative interpretations are available for people with disabilities who often feel as though they are the victims of wanton pronouncements and are powerless to respond to the God-is-on-your-side clichés.

In the ambiguities of these two stories from the gospels of Mark and John, our exploration offers powerful alternatives to the views that disability is a sign of faithlessness, that it is a sign of evil or caused by sin, and that suffering is a sign of God's will. Healing stories, nonetheless, will continue to be problematic for many people until disability is affirmed as an ordinary part of being human. Elizabeth Hastings (1995), who was Australia's first disability discrimination commissioner, offers a somewhat tongue-in-cheek but highly pertinent observation here:

> . . . with all the respect due to the ten lepers, the various possessed, and the sundry blind, lame, and deaf faithful of scripture, I reckon people who have disabilities may have been better off for the last two thousand years if Our Lord had not created quite so many miraculous cures but occasionally said, "your life is perfect as it is given to you–go ye and find its purpose and meaning," and to the onlookers, "this disability is an ordinary part of human being, go ye and create the miracle of a world free of discrimination." Which, of course, He did.

Rather than emphasizing the 'specialness' of people with disabilities, which leads to the knee-jerk response of damage-perpetuating clichés, the ordinariness of everyday life, notwithstanding the associated difficulties, needs to be constantly proclaimed and recognized by the church. The church would do well to articulate a theology that affirms and values people for who they are as part of God's good creation. As Betenbaugh (1992) says:

> Most reasonable people have long since abandoned the previously-held beliefs that being born black or female are signs of stigma, of being punished or cursed or forsaken by God. We are, slowly, making progress in reaching the same conclusion with gay and lesbian persons, but only as science moves ahead of us with discoveries that gender identity may be of biological origin and not a matter of choice, a "purely" psychological issue. Still lagging is the pronouncement of the same explicit understanding for those who are disabled. (p. 25)

The earlier contention was that the God-is-on-your-side clichés run the unacceptably high risk of alienating people with disabilities and their families from the very faith tradition that is called to be an instrument of reconciliation. It is timely to offer some alternative pastoral responses which acknowledge the grief and trauma, and which pro-actively support people in their search for meaning and connections with Christian faith. This is the 'in-between' place and time Pickard (1998) refers to: the verandah, from which Christian communities in Australia are invited and challenged to look with new eyes at the disempowering language used, and to listen with new ears to the stories of people with disabilities.

Honoring and respecting a person's lived experience are of paramount importance. Rather than offering a thoughtless and dismissive cliché, pastoral care best begins by listening intently to the person's story: to their struggles, hopes and fears. Historically, people with disabilities have not given voice to these, as they have been at the receiving end of charitable and paternalistic actions. But the winds of a sea change are blowing, albeit gently at times, as people are increasingly claiming their rightful place within all sectors of the community.

People with disabilities want to be heard; to have their voices considered with authority. Conversations need to be provoked by pastoral questions such as *What do you believe about this experience–about who you are?*; *Where is God in this for you?*; *Does it make sense to you?*; or *How does your journey/experience of faith help or hinder you in your current situation?* Newell (2002) asserts this also when he observes that:

> Comparatively little literature in the area of pastoral theology is actually written by people who consciously identify themselves as having a disability . . . we contend that the constant, mainstream presence of people with disabilities within the pastoral theological discussions surrounding the nature of and response to disability is critical . . . if we listen to the voices of people with disabilities, our theological understandings will be challenged and our pastoral responses sharpened and made more faithful. (Newell & Gillespie, 2002, p. 101)

Part of the sea change referred to is the increasing recognition that the lived experience of people with disabilities may indeed be a gift and comfort to other people, rather than something to be objectified and exorcised. Gillespie's (Newell & Gillespie, 2002) personal experience powerfully illustrates this:

> My understanding of my disability is that it is an intrinsic part of me. Imagine that I hold up my hand in front of you. Further, imagine that I say the front is valuable but the back has to go. It would be very obvious that this was not only impossible but also illogical. Here, the back of my hand is my psychosis; the front is the creativity, sensitivity and intelligence that attach to it. Even the psychotic experience has its value: I can stand next to the bereaved, the lonely, the stigmatised, the poor, the marginalised, the mad, the unheard, the rejected and the unloved, and truly convey by the warmth of my contact, my compassion and understanding. I do not need to judge or to disempower by assuming they cannot

find their own solutions. This is truly my greatest gift, and I have it because of my disability and the experience that has come with it. (p. 103)

In my own experience of road trauma and some years of physical recovery,
I am aware that it has become an intrinsic part of me, and, similarly, it shapes
my response of compassion and care for others. Part of that recovery included
others inviting me to share the story as I was ready and able, culminating in a
specially devised Celebration of Healing liturgy with friends and family seven
years after the event. A major pastoral issue in my own situation of disability
was an appreciation for people who recognized the impact of shock, and who
also knew, without trite explanations, that personal meaning would unfold
with time. Being 'companioned' on that journey with little, and not so little,
acts of kindness was more important than empty clichés.

Gaventa (1997) offers a foundational fourfold ministry response, the first
being that of pastoral care as companionship, as presence; pastoral care as an
act of incarnation: to be there at crucial and critical times (pp. 1-24). It is being
there in the times of transition when the necessary practical responses are required and the impact of the disability or impairment are more likely to raise
questions of meaning. It is being there without the expectation of having to
have the answers, but, rather, to listen and hear the lamentations, the anger, the
joy, the dreams and the frustrations. Such a non-anxious pastoral presence and
response which invites ministry to each other is poignantly captured by Bill
Williams (1998), a theologian with cystic fibrosis, who died in 1998:

> If we disappear from your sight, it may be because our courage failed.
> We decided not to burden you, and ourselves, with our presence.

But I've been with people who are not made anxious by my brokenness, and
I've seen the difference. It is, in fact, the best definition of ministry I have ever
heard; I nearly wept when I heard it, it so defined what I needed. Engrave this
upon your forehead, if you would wish to do good:

> *Ministry is a non-anxious presence.*

> You can tell such grace by its care, by its attentive ear, by its pace. When
> it reaches out to heal you, it is to give relief to you, not itself–and when it
> prays with you, it lets you declare your own burdens, rather than declar-
> ing what it finds burdensome about you . . . (p. 32)

The second of Gaventa's (1997) pastoral responses is that of guidance,
and being one who is acquainted with grief. In hearing the questions and as-
pirations, its emphasis is on helping people discover their own answers to

theological and spiritual issues. Earlier discussion touched on many of these theological issues of healing, faithfulness and sin. In addition, the issue of a person's disability as something that 'God has chosen for them,' and therefore part of God's will, is well dealt with by Pailin (1992, pp. 77-85). He considers the argument that according to God's will as Creator, disability is justifiable as a test of character. What is fundamentally wrong with this view is that God is depicted as behaving in a malevolent manner, and that many people become completely crushed by their life circumstances—hardly the stuff of a loving and caring parent.

As a guide, the pastoral carer is one who shares in the person's wrestling with these questions and issues and who is able to carefully and sensitively appropriate the life, death and resurrected experience of Christ. The pastoral care starts with the brokenness of God, and recognizes that disability and any sorrow or suffering which accompanies it is part of our common humanity. In the listening, without presuming or assuming, Gaventa points out that in the midst of their struggle many individuals and families are also full of life and joy and are able to recognize the blessings in their lives.

The third element of Gaventa's effective pastoral care in ministry with people with disabilities is that of shepherding, or, in modern parlance, advocacy. The shepherd of today is one who is prepared to go through the highs and lows, has a "rod and staff to comfort," helps to find a way through the wilderness of services and red tape, and has the audacity to celebrate "in the presence of my enemies" (Psalms 23). In keeping with the motifs from the image of shepherd in Psalm 23, the final one, dwelling in the house of the Lord forever, evokes powerful gifts of hospitality and sanctuary to the stranger. Such practical advocacy and welcome offers a powerful embrace for people who perhaps have low or non-existent expectations of pastoral care.

Steele (1994), writing of his daughter's experience with a rare musculoskeletal disease, cautions that in the laudable and necessary push for more accessible public and community facilities, we risk creating further barriers of human alienation. He and his family constantly feel that they are not 'strangers in a foreign land,' as the Bible calls travelers and resident aliens, but strangers in their own land, and thus, strangers indeed. Without a thorough change in the debilitating attitudes of heartless indifference and condescending pity, people labeled by disability will continue to be strangers in their own land. Steele (1994) also insists that hospitality and welcome are about more than stairs: it is about genuine respect and affection, which he has seen in the eyes of his daughter's physician who relates to her in many respects like a friend. It is this distinctive and positive gaze which people with disabilities need to receive from pastoral care. Friendship stands as a paradigm of pastoral care in need of further exploration, and I will offer some thoughts on this later in this article.

The fourth element of Gaventa's response is one of community building and empowerment of the 'Body' to care and offer support to each other. He asserts that this is too often a neglected pastoral skill in an age that focuses on individualism and one-to-one pastoral care. In the myriad ways that any congregation supports each other, it is especially important that people with disabilities and families are not left to wage the same battle for inclusion that they engage in for the other six days of the week. Involvement and equal opportunities for leadership in all areas of congregational life are powerful messages of acceptance, friendship and God's unconditional love. This applies not only in the receiving of support but also in the giving of support to others.

The pastoral implications of giving and receiving within the church are profound for people traditionally on the receiving end. How do we interpret Jesus' words, "It is more blessed to give than to receive?" Does this imply the receiver is not blessed, or that they are of lesser worth because they are the recipients? Is this about able-bodied people giving to people with disabilities so that the givers can feel good about themselves? The context within which Jesus' words are quoted is one of a call to support the 'weak.' Whether or not we subscribe to the notion that people with disabilities are 'weak,' the call, nonetheless, is one of mutual support and interdependence. I agree wholeheartedly with van Dongen-Garrad (1983), who argues persuasively for a renewed emphasis on the mutuality of giving and receiving:

> If giving promotes a person's sense of identity, participation and community, and discourages a sense of individual isolation, then giving would seem to be even more important for the disabled person than for the able-bodied person. We have seen that one of the ways in which a recipient can avoid being stigmatised or placed in the power of the giver is by becoming a giver also. (p. 84)

This was highlighted earlier with Gillespie's (Newell & Gillespie, 2002) reference to her ability to give the gift of compassion and understanding, which she claims arises directly from her experience of psychosis. As Betenbaugh (1992) further explores the pastoral implications of giving and receiving, she poses powerful observations for the church to grapple with:

> The person who gives is perceived to have more power and prestige than the person who receives. If one is under an obligation to another, then that person can only be "freed" by giving a service in return. Our culture values altruism, and the church further values it. We need to repeat anew the proclamation often found in Genesis and the Psalms, that to receive a gift is to receive the giver. The recipient is then understood to bless the

giver, even as he or she is blessed by the gift. Is this not at the root of our understanding of the Eucharist? (p. 30)

The issue of friendship as a paradigm of pastoral care is useful here, as pastoral care can run the risk of becoming a situation in which one person is the giver or provider giving to another, the receiver. The receiver is seen as having particular needs and that is the motivation for the care provided by the giver. There is nothing whatsoever to condemn in this. I wonder, however, in the light of Betenbaugh's and van Dongen-Garrad's observations, whether this particular motive and form of response have always been the most appropriate, or most complete, with people with disabilities?

In the previous consideration of the power dynamic in the giving-receiving relationship, it has historically been skewed in the direction of the person with a disability being the recipient of pastoral care. I wish to make some observations about friendship in the context of a caring community, which demands consideration as an additional pastoral response to the others mentioned in this paper. Gillespie found healing in caring relationships with two chaplains who offered friendship as opposed to distant professional relationships (Newell & Gillespie, 2002). Swinton (2000) also argues that:

> In a world that flees from pain and stigmatises suffering . . . the church [must] retrieve its fundamental identity as a passionate community that cares with the fervour of God and reveals that care in and through the precious gift of friendship. (p. 159)

In the New Testament, Jesus is referred to as a 'friend' on only two occasions; however, they are most important to the message of Jesus. In the Gospel of Luke we read: "The Son of Man has come eating and drinking, and you say, 'Behold a glutton and a drunkard, a friend of tax collectors and sinners!'" (Luke 7:34). Moltmann (1978) believes that the inner motivation for this striking friendship with people who are considered to be on the fringes of society lies in Jesus' celebration of the messianic feast of God's kingdom every time he eats and drinks with them (pp. 55-56). In combining affection and respect, he becomes their friend because of his joy in their common freedom–God's future. In the Gospel of John, we read:

> No-one has greater love than this, to lay down one's life for one's friends. You are my friends if you do what I command you. I do not call you servants any longer, because the servant does not know what the master is doing: but I have called you friends. (John 15:13-15a)

Here the sacrifice of one's life is the highest form of love, which manifests itself as friendship. The switch from being servants to being friends is most significant for the relationship between Jesus and the disciples. Moltmann believes that in the fellowship of Jesus, they now experience him in his innermost nature as 'Friend' (1978, p. 57). Open friendship becomes the bond in their fellowship, and, most significantly, becomes their vocation in a society still dominated by relationships of masters and servants.

In conclusion, this article has examined the God-is-on-your-side clichés, and revealed that upon close examination, they do not hold up at all well as caring pastoral responses. For some they may be a part of conversation about a person's situation. However, it is doubtful that many people would be reassured by such a limited Christian interpretation of God's care for them. Exegeses of the Marcan and Johannine texts reveal a degree of complexity, ambiguity and uncertainty behind some of the healing stories attributed to Jesus' ministry.

Hence, the God-is-on-your-side clichés examined in this article are trite and superficial in spite of their good intent. It is proposed that some of them could be interpreted as 'God-is-against-me' clichés. There are rarely easy explanations as to why people suffer. Popular sayings that reinforce God's association with suffering are among the poorest of pastoral responses.

Clichés such as these perpetuate the sense of victimhood and the collusion of God in the person's destiny, leaving little space to believe in anything other than a predetermined future. Alternative pastoral responses explored herein offer people with disabilities a sense of companionship, a place of being listened to, of challenge and nurture, to discern the meaning of their lived experience in affirming and mutually beneficial support systems and friendships. Sometimes too, when there are no easy answers, or jaundiced theology, it means having someone to sit with in that 'in-between' place, like the Australian verandah, in silence. In these pastoral responses, it is hoped that a person's move towards wholeness and reconciliation with God, self and community is nurtured and blessed.

REFERENCES

Betenbaugh, H. (1992). *A theology of disability*. Dallas, Texas: Perkins School of Theology.
Eiesland, N. L. (1994). *The disabled God: Toward a liberatory theology of disability*. Nashville: Abingdon Press.
Eiesland, N. L., & Saliers, D. E. (Eds.) (1998). *Human disability and the service of God: Reassessing religious practices*. Nashville: Abingdon Press.
Fulcher, G. (1989). *Disabling policies?* London: Falmer Press.

Fullwood, D., & Cronin, P. (1986). *Facing the crowd: Managing other people's insensitivities to your disabled child.* Melbourne: Royal Victorian Institute for the Blind.

Gaventa, W. C. (1997). Pastoral care with people with disabilities and their families: An adaptable module for introductory courses. In *Thematic conversations regarding disability within the framework of courses of worship, Scripture and pastoral care.* Dayton: National Council of Churches Committee on Disabilities.

Grant, C. C. (1998). Reinterpreting the healing narratives. In N. L. Eiesland & D. E. Saliers (Eds.), *Human disability and the service of God: Reassessing religious practice* (pp. 78-87). Nashville: Abingdon Press.

Hastings, E. (1995). *Include me in.* Paper delivered to the NSW Uniting Church in Australia, Synod of 1995.

Moltmann, J. (1978). *The open Church.* London: SCM Press.

Newell, C., & Gillespie, F. (2002). Narrative, psychiatric disability, and pastoral care: Towards a richer theology of disability. In C. Newell (Ed.), *Exclusion and embrace: Conversations about spirituality and disability* (pp. 201-207). Papers from the Third National Conference on Spirituality and Disability, 2001. Melbourne: UnitingCare Victoria.

Pailin, D. A. (1992). *A gentle touch: From a theology of handicap to a theology of human being.* London: SPCK.

Pickard, S. (1998). The view from the verandah: Gospel and spirituality in an Australian setting. *St. Marks Review, Winter.*

Senior, D. (1995). Beware of the Canaanite woman: Disability and the Bible. In Marilyn Bishop (Ed.), *Religion and disability: Essays in Scripture, theology, and ethics* (pp. 1-25). Kansa City: Sheed & Ward.

Steele, R. B. (1994). Accessibility or hospitality? Reflections and experiences of a father and theologian. *Journal of Religion in Disability & Rehabilitation, 1:1* (pp. 11-26). Haworth Pastoral Press.

Swinton, J. (2000). *From Bedlam to Shalom: Towards a practical theology of human nature, interpersonal relationships, and mental health care.* Peter Lang: New York.

Tacey, D. (1995). *The edge of the sacred: Transformation in Australia.* Melbourne: Harper Collins.

Tiffany, F. C., & Ringe, S. H. (1996). *Biblical interpretation: A roadmap.* Nashville: Abingdon Press.

Van Dongen-Garrad, J. (1983). *Invisible barriers: Pastoral care with physically disabled people.* London: SPCK.

Williams, B. (1998). *Naked before God: The return of a broken disciple.* Harrisburg, PA: Morehouse.

Disability, Ethics, and Biotechnology: Where Are We Now?

Jayne Clapton, RN, BA, PhD

SUMMARY. This paper was originally presented in memory of Jennifer Fitzgerald, as an address at a Queensland conference. Jennifer Fitzgerald was a lawyer and writer working in the 1990s with Queensland Advocacy Incorporated (QAI), an independent, community-based systems advocacy and legal advocacy organisation for people with disability in Queensland, Australia. As QAI's first bioethics advocacy worker, Jenny insightfully identified the threats posed by areas of biotechnology, for people with disability. Her works include a collection of papers on ethical issues facing people with disability, and "Include Me In: Disability Rights and the Law in Queensland" (1994). She was also a published participant of the first conference on Disability, Health and Spirituality held in Brisbane in 1996. *[Article copies available for a fee from The Haworth Document Delivery Service: 1-800-HAWORTH. E-mail address: <docdelivery@haworthpress.com> Website: <http://www.Haworth Press.com> © 2004 by The Haworth Press, Inc. All rights reserved.]*

KEYWORDS. Ethics, disability, biotechnology, bioethics

Jayne Clapton is Lecturer, School of Human Services, Griffith University.

Address correspondence to: Dr. Jayne Clapton, School of Human Services, Logan Campus, Griffith University, University Drive, Meadowbrook, 4131, Queensland, Australia (E-mail: J.Clapton@mailbox.gu.edu.au).

[Haworth co-indexing entry note]: "Disability, Ethics, and Biotechnology: Where Are We Now?" Clapton, Jayne. Co-published simultaneously in *Journal of Religion, Disability & Health* (The Haworth Pastoral Press, an imprint of The Haworth Press, Inc.) Vol. 8, No. 1/2, 2004, pp. 21-31; and: *Voices in Disability and Spirituality from the Land Down Under: Outback to Outfront* (ed: Christopher Newell, and Andy Calder) The Haworth Pastoral Press, an imprint of The Haworth Press, Inc., 2004, pp. 21-31. Single or multiple copies of this article are available for a fee from The Haworth Document Delivery Service [1-800-HAWORTH, 9:00 a.m. - 5:00 p.m. (EST). E-mail address: docdelivery@haworthpress.com].

http://www.haworthpress.com/web/JRDH
© 2004 by The Haworth Press, Inc. All rights reserved.
Digital Object Identifier: 10.1300/J095v8n01_03

It is indeed an honor and a privilege for me to have been asked to deliver this Inaugural Jennifer Fitzgerald Memorial Address and to explore a topic to which Jenny made such a significant contribution.

I want to begin with a story. In April this year, our family received a beautiful book from a friend who lives in Adelaide. The book, from the Art Gallery of South Australia, was of a recent exhibition of the drawings and paintings created in two voyages around Australia at the beginning of the nineteenth century. Underpinning the significance of the exhibition is the story of an historic encounter in February 1802 when the two ships, one British and one French, met in the Southern Ocean at what is now called Encounter Bay, near the present site of Adelaide (Radford, 2002).

The British ship, the *Investigator*, was captained by Matthew Flinders. He was accompanied by scientists interested in the biological and anthropological findings, which were interpreted and represented by two artists: Ferdinand Bauer, one of the greatest natural history artists of all time, and William Westall, the first and one of the finest of Australia's nineteenth century landscape artists (Thomas, 2002).

On the other hand, the French ship, le *Géographe*, was captained by Nicolas Baudin. The scientists on this voyage were supported by Charles-Alexandre Lesueur, who created some of the world's most beautiful watercolors of exotic sea creatures, and Nicolas-Martin Petit, who is recognized as having painted some of the most sensitive and accurate depictions of Australian Aboriginal people (Thomas, 2002).

However, the Encounter Bay experience had deeper significance. The two voyages also represented two rival imperial cultures which at that time were at war (Radford, 2002). In fact, it was only through the two captains' demonstrated commitment to a "commonwealth of learning" that a peaceful and sharing encounter was achieved (Radford, 2002, p. 6).

In such a geopolitical context, Britain and France were the two richest and most powerful countries in the world, with their imperial power enhanced by empirical observation serving both scientific and political objectives. In other words, not only were the four artists busily engaged in sketching the plants, animals, native inhabitants and coastal landscapes of one of the last undiscovered continents on earth, but they were also the key participants of colonizing endeavors. This was at a time when the world was conceived as being a finite, knowable entity: in its mapping, in the systems of classification, and in its naming processes (Thomas 2002). Therefore, the search for new shipping routes and continents would provide increased opportunities for trade and more foreign lands to colonize, and through emerging scientific knowledge, new opportunities would arise for an increased demand for markets and resources (Thomas, 2002). Thinking that the chaos of nature could be tamed, an imperial gaze was thus cast upon the careful dissection and visual representation of flora and fauna. This also encapsulated depictions and interpretations of the native inhabitants, which were all surveyed primarily from the coastal edge of a new continent (Thomas, 2002).

Many of you may be wondering why I am telling this story–a story that is surprising even for me, given that up until the last five years or so, my knowledge and observation of southern exploration was restricted to the sighting of Victorian number-plates coming to Queensland for winter.

However, the story does have analogous significance for the rest of this address. For instance, as Sarah Thomas (2002) states two centuries later, the frontiers of exploration have shifted–in one direction away from earth altogether, into space, and in another, into the realms of microscopy, exploring genes, cells and other building blocks of life. Today the views of these new frontiers which are captured by the latest imaging technologies have the same capacity to inspire wonder (and, I would add, capital) as the exotic watercolors first seen by Europeans after the Flinders and Baudin expeditions (Thomas, 2002). These technologies and the emergence of new knowledge are therefore enmeshed under the broad term *biotechnology* in this genetic era.

However, I argue that today, like then, such 'voyages of discovery' undertaken by 'frontier explorers' are not just depicted in the same language but also loaded with a similar political agenda of discovery and commerce. For instance, relationships between science and economics have seen research become the medium of the new shipping route providing a pathway supported by partnerships between universities, government and venture-capital investors. These, in turn, have created a highly competitive, politically priority-driven research agenda which is now privileged over previous individualized curiosity-driven research. Also, in this change, the focus of research has shifted to seeking causes rather than merely describing correlations or offering explanations (Suzuki, 2001; Commonwealth of Australia, 1999). Consequently, such a context offers new (even unanticipated) choices demanding decisions in which an encounter with the practice of ethics for guidance is deemed inevitable (Peterson 2001). It is the *nature* of this encounter, then, which is predominantly scrutinized. For instance, to what degree does the encounter between two imperial disciplines such as biotechnology and ethics represent an encounter between warring parties, or that of two components sharing the commonwealth of knowledge in the name of the advancement of knowledge?

According to Sloan (2000), the current biotechnological context poses questions about the moral limitations on the technological manipulation of life, about the definition of individual and social goods, and about the nature of the human person. A significant question emerges for attention: to what degree does an encounter between biotechnology and ethics also represent a somewhat concealed agenda of control and colonization?

At this point, Alice Dreger's (2000) illumination of a colonial agenda of biotechnology is useful. She describes how the American political context depicted the Human Genome Project as a 'dramatic morality play' (p. 158). In this 'play,' she also describes how scientists have been depicted as frontier explorers on journeys of discovery; with the discovered territory then claimed and mapped as a road map to good health. Dreger (2000) identifies a further agenda based on the intensity of the subsequent claims that it would be *immoral* or *unethical* not to carry on with the project because a moral imperative of seeking 'good' is paramount. And, of course, such a progressive agenda then culminates in engaging in real estate practices of commodifying and trading the territory for economic gain (Dreger, 2000).

With the biotechnological agenda seeking *good*, the dominant underlying ethics are premised, therefore, upon *utilitarian* approaches which seek the greatest good for the greatest number–a *good* that also includes the utilization of economic imperatives to create *cost benefits* and to *relieve* and *control* societal burden.

In this moral context of the genetic era, powerful disciplinary partnerships are formed, for example, between science, medicine, law, philosophy, ethics, and politics. The practitioners are not only seen as virtuous pioneers who are given societal authority as the custodians of the *good*, but are also acknowledged as salvationists from the *bad*. By using language and tropes of hunting the 'bad' genes (Dreger, 2000), this constructed moral imperative both likens the agenda to the rationale of a 'just war' and necessarily depicts the representatives of the bad genes as morally harmful.

Some deep implications and questions therefore emerge. If the use of biotechnology is legitimated in the name of the *good*, we need to ask then, what represents *good*? And conversely, what represents *not good*, or, in fact, *bad*? As well, we must explore who has the power to decide these, and why. And, importantly, who are rendered voiceless in this construction?

I contend that these are deep questions which are not simply answered by focusing on the nature of the encounter between imperial disciplines such as biotechnology and ethics. Rather they can only be addressed by shifting our scrutiny to the *quality of the images* portraying the subjects of the imperial gaze and political agenda. One such set of images that must be explored is how people with disability are perceived.

Sadly, though, the significance of the imaging of people with disability which I am referring to has received very little public attention, let alone reaching the arenas of ethical deliberations, public policy making or even public debates. As a matter of fact, one could even wonder to what degree the dazzle and luster of shining potential dollar signs shimmering from the surface of political initiatives in biotechnology actually blind us from seeing the subjects, or perhaps 'objects,' presupposed within it.

Through European history, perceptions and motivations, Indigenous Australians were perceived, two hundred years ago, as inferior *others*. However, in this contemporary era, we recognize the inadequacy of the objective representations of the Australian Aboriginal people, depicted from the distance by artists on voyages of discovery (Morphy, 2002). We have come to acknowledge how in such images, the artists only depicted the morphology of Aboriginal people, and therefore failed to capture the real lived ecological accounts of people living in community with each other. Moreover, we have now rescinded actions made under the dictum of *terra nullius*, which denied political or moral rights of Indigenous Australians to belong.

People with disability have historically been portrayed by the dominating disciplines of science, medicine and philosophy as deficit beings, whereby their status of humanity and personhood have been continually questioned. Therefore, in such a colonizing context which preferences a reductionist and even unitary way of being human, those seen as different or, more likely, potentially different, and thus scaled as inferior, are in peril and at risk of eradication and extermination. For example, along with the creation of new diagnostic procedures such as genetic testing and diagnosis, as well as advanced foetal screening techniques and more sophisticated Assisted Reproductive Technologies (ART), not only has knowledge expanded, but more choices are available also. These are offered in the context of autonomy and freedom to choose not only what humans make up the social world but also why some should not become part of it. In fact, the predominant critique offered by disability rights activists is to question biotechnology as a eugenic process for the implicit power within it to negatively discriminate against people and potential people with disability (see, for example, Parens & Asch, 2000; Vehmas, 1999; Shakespeare, 1998). Not surprisingly though, such an accusation is rejected by scientists and clinicians alike who defend their practices as being based upon ethical principles of seeking the good and offering beneficence and compassion to those who suffer or will potentially suffer (see, for example, Gillon, 2001; Gillott, 2001).

I argue, though, that to engage in such a polarized debate merely presents a smokescreen to ethical deliberation. What must be intrinsic to the discussion are not the outcomes but the reasoning and discursive constructions within the presenting images. In biotechnological contexts (as, incidentally, in other current public policy concerns such as medical insurance and public liability insurance), people with disability are perceived as suffering, dependent, useless, and burdensome beings who would be incapable of happiness and moral competency. Therefore, preventative, eliminating or compensatory interventions should be enacted to reduce suffering and minimize harm (Reinders, 2000). The double effect, if you like, of such actions is that people with disability become undesirable and risk irrelevance in the public arena.

But why is this so? In previous research, I have identified that such images are embedded in a dominant conjunction constituted by two contributing elements. These are *bioethics* as traditional medical ethics, and *disability* conceptualized as a personal tragedy.

Bioethics as traditional medical ethics is based upon traditional ethical perspectives and principles, which privilege a particular understanding of personhood. The presumed person (or potential person) is a prototypical disembodied person who is typically a propertied male, characterized by independence and the presence of rationality and reason. Those who represent *anomalous others* to this are only morally included if they can assimilate to similar characteristics. In ethics literature, of course, such a view is often questioned, and alternative ways of 'doing ethics' are presented. However, many people with disability, particularly with intellectual disability, regardless of different ethics methodologies, remain continually subjected both to moral exclusion and the betrayal of ethics as a discipline, to protect them.

When disability is perceived as a personal tragedy, impairment and disability are conflated as an observable trait. Socio-ethical identities are thus constructed from biologically deficit understandings based on labels, limitation and loss of the 'individual' (with the problem). The focus, then, is on the alleviation of presumed suffering and unhappiness, as well as monitoring the *costs* of dependency and burden. Hence, expert intervention is required, which is usually formulated and coordinated within a medical model. Although the medical model has offered compassion and care for some, it has also been problematic for many others.

However, the tragedy view of disablement has now been subject to critique for over 35 years. Some of the more contemporary critiques shift the focus of disablement away from seemingly problematic and dysfunctional individuals to the structures of an excluding and oppressing society. Through the enactment of disability rights, for example, access to social structures such as education, employment, and community citizenship has been fought for through political processes that challenge discrimination and exclusion.

Unfortunately, such a significant paradigmatic shift has remained elusive in contemporary ethical considerations around disability and biotechnology. A glance at any guiding codes of ethics, for instance, will confirm this view. Although living people with disability are recognized as beings to be respected, the status of potential persons–or, more accurately, non-persons–remains as potential sources of harm and 'not-good' (see, for example, Queensland Government, 2001). Technologies and procedures performed on this basis are rarely questioned. For many people with disability, this betrayal is akin to processes of re-colonization.

The Australian Aboriginal peoples treated their colonizers with suspicion because of their continuing experience of intrusion, fear, domination, oppression, separation, violence and sexual exploitation. Likewise, people with disability and their advocates are suspicious of the biotechnological agenda for the similar reasons attributed to a society that perpetuates moral exclusion of some of its members.

Significantly then, the two elements–bioethics as traditional medical ethics, and disability as personal tragedy–predominate and then become conjointly responsible for two dominant discourses which image disability in biotechnology. These, I name "discourses of *tragedy* and *catastrophe*" (Clapton, in press).

A discourse of tragedy is underpinned by the meaning of *tragedy*, which in this context is seen as an unhappy event or series of events in real life, with disastrous or sorrowful conclusions (according to the *Shorter Oxford Dictionary*, 1992). This discourse is characteristically enacted in the private arena, such as a clinical encounter, and therefore, the stakeholders are most likely restricted to such a site. Issues of suffering and harm are thus presented, confronted and deliberated upon through private decision-making processes, often with professional assistance. The quality of information is important, but in this context, it is most likely framed from a 'personal tragedy' perspective; whereby people (or potential people) with disability are viewed as deficient individuals who will invariably suffer and cause distress and burden. Ethically, the privacy of such a context is afforded utmost respect as deliberations about personal harm are negotiated. I would argue, then, that accusations of eugenic intentions do not have a place in this discursive construction. However, the degree to which alternative framings of disability (other than that of being a tragedy) are, or become, represented in such an encounter will remain the ongoing challenge for education and professional reflection. This is dependent, of course, on the imperative for the professionals involved to recognize the constraints of viewing disability only through such a deficit-focused medical model.

On the other hand, though, it is the discourse of catastrophe that is in urgent need of public attention and debate. In this context, an image of disability as *catastrophe* embraces a notion of *a sudden disaster due to the disruption of an established social order* (according to the *Shorter Oxford Dictionary*). What is at stake in this discursive construction is the 'health' of the society at large. The focus, then, is on how to develop and use different measures to protect such a society from any impending threats such as economic burden and non-productivity. In this public context, where disability is viewed as problematic and, hence, detrimental to societal wealth and well-being, scientists and clinicians of biotechnology are socially constructed and presented, usually with the support of the political arena, as virtuous pioneers and salvationists who carry the responsibility of creating not only better humans but also enhanced societies (Commonwealth of Australia, 1999). In such a context, we see a convergence between biotechnology and ethics, sharing a political intent of controlling their construction of *otherness*.

It becomes apparent that achieving this with dependency upon a utilitarian ethical framework is problematic. Ethics, rather than providing a safety net in ethical deliberations, acts complicitly within a colonizing agenda to render irrelevant some alternative, yet authenticating, accounts of the subjectivity of some of the 'objects' of the scientific endeavor. In this context, people such as those with disability have come to represent the undesirable way of being human, and are therefore denied the respect of potential personhood. In other words, in a social order which claims a universal subject which is normatively protected, those who differ from the norm and relegated to the inferior status of the 'not-right.' Other are also synonymously imaged as being 'not-good.' Having been constructed as harm-causing burdens and threats to families and society, the necessity to prevent, control or eradicate becomes paramount. To be able to achieve this with the gathering of wealth through a colonizing agenda is indeed a lucrative task.

This view, though, is contrary to meanings of burden as described by families. It is not their family *member* who is the burden. Rather, burden represents a correlation between their family *experiences* and inadequate financial and social support and resources offered by communities and governments (Dowling & Dolan, 2001). The concealed ethical challenge is to what degree such resources do or do not support a moral commitment that people with disability, being part of the wide scope of humanity, belong as *integral* members in society, rather than merely seen as an optional presence. Such a moral claim cannot be derived from ethics that promote people with disability objectively as deficit humans or non-persons. Instead, ethics that affirm *all* people as relational subjects capable of sharing mutual and respectful relationships with others must be embraced and promoted in biotechnological discussions.

Therefore, how ought we as members of society to respond to these ethical complexities? A response is not so much waiting to be found but, rather, to be recognized. It is to the character and contribution of Jenny Fitzgerald that we must now turn.

Jenny Fitzgerald was an insightful pioneering explorer. When she began writing about some of these challenges in the early 1990s, not only did she do so in isolation from the disability field who could not, at that point, recognize what was happening, but she also did so with courage, and even fearlessness at times, as she confronted the imperial powers dictating the emerging agenda. Very early, she recognized the powerful constructions of the images being portrayed, and set about challenging them in private discussions and also in public forums and debates. Her strength was to do this even when it meant, for her, experiences of pain and struggle.

Jenny Fitzgerald was an outstanding and wise scholar. Her writings depicted a deep capacity to cast an alternative gaze upon people with disability as relational subjects, and not merely as empirical objects. She articulated and pursued the rights of people with disability to be integral members of society, and she challenged the dominating values that not only denied the stories and silences of their lived experience but also their subjection to processes of oppression and injustice. In doing this, she set about utilizing forms of scholarship other than the predominant perspectives; insightfully creating opportunities for a more ethical response outside of established methods. This is exemplified, for instance, in her published paper presented at the 1996 Brisbane conference on Disability, Religion and Health, exploring the spiritual dimensions of disability. In that paper, Jenny highlighted how medical and evolving genetic models of disability serve to construct disability, and how society has legitimated responses of isolation, segregation and elimination. She also identified how such constructions define and confine the spirituality of people with disability, in terms of affecting the possibility of an integrated, interdependent and holistic view of the self and society. In other words, favoring a controlling mechanized and bureaucratic world view such as that promoted within biotechnology, she argued, will continue to suppress the freedom of people with disability to explore their spirituality and sense of being (Fitzgerald, 1997). It is significant even today that when she expressed wisdom in a context in which power was the dominant currency, Jenny did so, not by appeasing the elite, but from a profound understanding of the positioning of 'otherness' and by questioning the legitimacy of such a position.

And finally, Jenny Fitzgerald was my friend. It is indeed a great privilege for me to have shared a friendship with Jenny. The times that I journeyed with her, both academically and, later, personally, were rich and memorable. The sharing of knowledge, which we both enjoyed, culminated with our writing one of her last publications together (Clapton & Fitzgerald, 1997). Later, our sharing was to take more personal forms such as reflecting upon the fragility of life and death. The fact that Jenny is no longer here to contribute to these dense discussions is indeed our loss.

In conclusion then, as John Ralston Saul (2001) suggests in his latest book, *On Equlibrium*, the quality of ethics is not in acceptance or rejection of a point of view, but in the *quality of the consideration* given to it. Within the context of Disability, Ethics and Biotechnology, Jenny Fitzgerald gave us the opportunity to enrich that quality to where we are today. Where we go from here will depend on how much we see it as our responsibility to give her contribution due consideration.

REFERENCES

Clapton, J. (in press). Tragedy and catastrophe: Contentious discourses of ethics and disability. *Journal of Intellectual Disability Research.*

Clapton, J., & Fitzgerald, J. (1997). The history of disability: A history of otherness. *New Renaissance, 7* (1), 20-21, 31.

Commonwealth of Australia. (1999). The virtuous cycle: Working together for health and medical research. *Health and Medical Research Strategic Review.* Canberra: AGPS.

Dowling, M., & Dolan, L. (2001). Families with children with disabilities–Inequalities and the social model. *Disability & Society, 16* (1), pp. 21-35.

Dreger, A. (2000). Metaphors of morality in the Human Genome Project. In P. Sloan (Ed.), *Controlling our destinies* (pp. 155-184). Notre Dame, Indiana: University of Notre Dame Press.

Fitzgerald, J. (1997). Reclaiming the whole: Self, spirit, and society. *Disability and Rehabilitation, 19* (10), pp. 407-413.

Gillon, R. (2001). Is there a 'new ethics of abortion'? *Journal of Medical Ethics, 27,* Supplement, pp. 115-119.

Gillott, J. (2001). Screening for disability: A eugenic pursuit? *Journal of Medical Ethics, 27,* Supplement, II 121-II 123.

Morphy, H. (2002). Encountering aborigines. In S. Thomas (Ed.), *The encounter, 1802: Art of the Flinders and Baudin voyages* (pp. 148-175). Adelaide: Art Gallery of South Australia.

Parens, E., & Asch, A. (Eds.) (2000). *Prenatal testing and disability rights.* Washington DC: Georgetown University Press.

Peterson, J. (2001). *Genetic turning points: The ethics of human genetic intervention.* Grand Rapids, Michigan: William B. Eerdmans Pub. Co.

Queensland Government. (2001). *Code of ethical practice for biotechnology in Queensland: Advancement through safe and ethical science.* Brisbane: Queensland Government.

Radford, R. (2002). Foreword. In S. Thomas (Ed.), *The Encounter, 1802: Art of the Flinders and Baudin Voyages* (pp. 6-8). Adelaide: Art Gallery of South Australia.

Reinders, H. (2000). *The future of the disabled in liberal society: An ethical analysis.* Notre Dame, Indiana: University of Notre Dame Press.

Saul, J. R. (2001). *On equilibrium.* Ringwood, Vic.: Penguin Books.

Shakespeare, T. (1998). Choices and rights: Eugenics, genetics and disability equality. *Disability & Society, 13* (5), pp. 665-681.

Sloan, P. (2000). Preface. In P. Sloan (Ed.), *Controlling our destinies* (pp. xxii-xxx). Notre Dame, Indiana: University of Notre Dame Press.

Suzuki, D. (2001). Introduction: A geneticist's reflections on the new genetics. In R. Hindmarsh & G. Lawrence (Eds.), *Altered genes II* (pp. 1-8). Melbourne: Scribe Publications.

The Shorter Oxford Dictionary on Historical Principles (1992). Oxford: Clarendon Press.

Thomas, S. (Ed.). (2002). *The Encounter, 1802: Art of the Flinders and Baudin Voyages*. Adelaide: Art Gallery of South Australia.

Vehmas, S. (1999). Discriminative assumptions of utilitarian bioethics regarding individuals with intellectual disabilities. *Disability & Society, 14* (1), pp. 37-52.

"Believe That a Farther Shore Is Reachable from Here": Mapping Community as Moral Loving Journeying

Lorna Hallahan, BSW, Doctoral Candidate

SUMMARY. How do relationships become transformational for all of us? Asking why people with disability should bother with community, this paper explores the concept of *communio* as loving, moral journeying. Asking who shall travel with us, the paper also looks closely at the qualities of people who can be mobilized to bridge differences. In this way, community is seen as verb rather than noun, as praxis rather than goal, as activity rather than product, as participation rather than membership, as embarking rather than arriving, as fickle rather than fixed, as insecure rather than stitched up, as adventure rather than feat, as desire and disappointment rather than destination. And living thus, we can trek to that farther shore–vital and resilient community. *[Article copies available for a fee from The Haworth Document Delivery Service: 1-800-HAWORTH. E-mail address: <docdelivery@haworthpress.com> Website: <http://www.HaworthPress.com> © 2004 by The Haworth Press, Inc. All rights reserved.]*

Lorna Hallahan is Coordinator of the Disability and Spirituality Project, Flinders University Centre for Theology, Science and Culture, GPO 2100, Adelaide, South Australia 5001, Australia (E-mail: lorna.hallahan@flinders.edu.au).

[Haworth co-indexing entry note]: ""Believe That a Farther Shore Is Reachable from Here": Mapping Community as Moral Loving Journeying." Hallahan, Lorna. Co-published simultaneously in *Journal of Religion, Disability & Health* (The Haworth Pastoral Press, an imprint of The Haworth Press, Inc.) Vol. 8, No. 1/2, 2004, pp. 33-44; and: *Voices in Disability and Spirituality from the Land Down Under: Outback to Outfront* (ed: Christopher Newell, and Andy Calder) The Haworth Pastoral Press, an imprint of The Haworth Press, Inc., 2004, pp. 33-44. Single or multiple copies of this article are available for a fee from The Haworth Document Delivery Service [1-800-HAWORTH, 9:00 a.m. - 5:00 p.m. (EST). E-mail address: docdelivery@haworthpress.com].

http://www.haworthpress.com/web/JRDH
© 2004 by The Haworth Press, Inc. All rights reserved.
Digital Object Identifier: 10.1300/J095v8n01_04

KEYWORDS. Disability, spirituality, community development, communio

Let us give birth to the unexpected
So hope for a great sea change
On the far side of revenge
Believe that a farther shore
Is reachable from here

(Seamus Heaney, from *Cure of Troy*)

In the beginning is the relation, says Martin Buber (1958). I want to say that, also, in the middle and in the end is the relation. There is no entity called autonomy and no state called independence. So what's new? Talking about the significance of community for people with disability is a bit like a preacher having to breathe new and creative insights into the parable of the prodigal son, or a doctor advocating the value of nose wiping and hand washing in a child-care center. There is not really much that one can say that hasn't been tried before.[1]

Not only is it hard to find anything refreshing to say about community, but we are really talking about nurturing loving relationships amongst people, and love, also, is wearied. What could possibly revive it? F. E. Jeffers (1996), writing in the *Humanist*, puts the challenge this way:

> When the well-intentioned children of light admonish us to love one another, it is like the nutritionist advising us to consume healthy food. Such prescriptions are desirable, even necessary, for individual and societal well-being, but they are after-the-fact directives which do not take into account the complex internal histories of the persons to whom they are addressed. Loving is organic; to be able to love involves an internal understanding of one's relatedness, a felt connectedness to another person or to anything else external to the person experiencing the connection. (p. 21)

Quite so–we do not love on order. So first, a promise: I promise I won't mention 'community education' as the way to people's hearts.[2] Now a confession: I love solitude and I love households. I tend to avoid the public, even though I have a good liberal view that, generally, human beings tend towards the decent and away from deliberate evil. I like my relationships kind of cozy, supportive, encouraging, and all that. And even in this, I let myself down; I don't deal very well with animosity, anger or prolonged anguish in relationships. I'd like to be a person of enormous heart; a bold person with a capacity to reach both within myself and beyond myself to embrace the many people who I know are lonely. (Please don't get me wrong–I am not suggesting that all of your life's problems will be solved if, in generous mode, I am your best friend. For one thing, my life is not all that exciting!) The point is this: any talk about extending beyond the safe ground of existing connections is as much directed at me as it is at others. And knowing this, I also know that no amount of trying to convince me to be a better person is going to help. I had many years of dedicated goodness training that really taught me the skills of condescension. The barriers that I feel in welcoming strangers–and I mean really welcoming–seem to be more than moral failings. It is not so much a failure to do things right; it seems more like a failure to care and to love deeply enough.

The question remains–is there any way to people's hearts? Gabriel Marcel, the French Christian existentialist, made a distinction between a problem and a mystery. Gertrude MacIntyre (1997) describes it thus:

> A problem is outside you, and will be solved depending on the available technology and resources. A mystery lies within your inner dimensions as you interact with the outside world. Action in this field goes beyond simply solving problems. Community development becomes a mirror to oneself and window on the wider world. Sometimes you do not like what you see there, but the experience is always rewarding. (p. 10)[3]

I agree–sometimes I might not like what I see in this mysterious area of community development, and because of that, I believe the experience of exploring it can be rewarding.

First, community needs to be put in its place. It pops up everywhere, and it's supposed to reassure me. I have some fairly grave doubts about the many claims made for community in the lives of poor, lonely, and rejected people. It seems that the uglier our attitudes, the more vocal our claims about community. Now this is the only time the hard-line postmodernist will agree with me: we can deconstruct community. We all have our own bugbears, but I want to attack six main lies about community:

1. Sentimental sludge aimed at enlisting my support for some pretty foul things such as thinking that turning away or indefinitely detaining asylum seekers is evidence of how Australia is a community; that is, the lie that community emerges from scapegoating the outsiders.
2. Deceit aimed at concealing an increasing shift away from government concern in the lives of certain citizens. MacIntyre (1997), reflecting on the multiple meanings of community and the many motivations to com-

munity development, gives this vivid historical insight: "Community development has often been a child of hard times, and this is one reason for its increasing popularity among governments as a way of handling increasing expectations in a time of limited resources.[4] (p. 1)

3. The Garden of Eden myth that community had a golden age just at the time we had incredibly high rates of institutionalization or imprisonment of all sorts of people who couldn't submit to the reign of suburban life.

4. The Heaven on Earth myth that we are growing into a sort of multicultural funfest that brings us all in from the cold and exuberantly celebrates difference as a source of enrichment, at the same time that we celebrate the emergence of technologies that will reduce the burden of aged and disabled people upon those of us who are young, fit, aspiring workers.

5. Charity and condescension, masquerading as compassion, care and mutuality, demanding humble gratitude.

6. Marketing (buy our product, share our values, join with everyone else who believes in nation, family, and Microsoft!) aimed at building up groups of all too eager consumers of products usually made elsewhere by people who have no hope of ever owning the thing they make.[5]

If 'community' is such a corrupt notion and, in its ideal state, so remote, why bother with it? In the knowledge that, so often, turning our faces towards the communities around us brings rejection and dejection, aren't people with disability better off relinquishing the desire for connection that honors, cares about, and expands their lives and their knowledge of self? Why set people up for more disappointment? Given that relationships bring pain along with the promise of pleasure, how can relationships become transformational for all of us?[6] Can anything be rescued or created here?

It is important to keep this skepticism going and, certainly, to apply the same filters to what I have to say, but not forever. Why?–because deconstruction can end up simply describing the exercise of power; especially the deceptive power of language. Judgements must be made. Inequality breeds horrible things in people's lives: tragedy, resentment and rejection, to name but three. These things must be challenged at every possible point. I suggest we proceed with a dialectic of skepticism and commitment. It is possible to be constructive by being both appreciative and critical of the range of traditions available to us from community development and ecclesiology; theology and disability studies; history and psychology.

It is always worthwhile to relentlessly pursue ways that people can become justly engaged in each other's lives. The choice is quite stark really. This is the way Kenny Fries (1997) puts it in *Staring Back: The Disability Experience from the Inside Out*:

> Throughout history, those who live with disabilities have been isolated in institutions, experimented upon, exterminated. We have been silenced by those who didn't want to hear what we have to say. We have also been silenced by our own fear, the fear that if we told our stories people would say: "See, it isn't worth it. You would be better off dead." (p. 1)

It is precisely and simply because people with disability would not be better off dead that we can remain dedicated in our efforts to resist exclusion and to strive for embrace. And to this we can add some insights from those who have encouraged others to move beyond the claustrophobia of familiarity, and those who have sought to extend their sphere of relationships to foster the prospects of threatened others.[7]

Schratz and Walker (in MacIntyre, 1997) point out four dimensions of human existence, around which community development and any effort at bringing about change revolves:

> Closeness, distance, continuity, and change are . . . arms of a cross pulling in four different directions. Closeness requires familiarity, longing for love, social contact, harmony, and commitment. Distance involves a quest for difference, individualism, freedom, autonomy. The tensions in meeting these two opposing demands are played out in time and space in communities. Continuity depends on order, planning, rules, power arrangements, control, while change focuses on the lure of the unknown, the new, escapes from the familiar, alteration to established patterns, spontaneity. . . . Closeness and distance, continuity, and change are not polar opposites. They are phenomena that can be presented as the ends of a spectrum. Everyone requires close relationships with others to flourish–and time alone. Everyone seeks stability and security–and also opportunities for change. Community development seeks to balance the contrasting needs for stability and security and those focused on change. Thus the process always has a highly ambiguous feel to it.[8] (Cited in MacIntyre, 1997, p. 5)

Within the context of this ambiguity, I make two contributions that can speak to this need for closeness amongst those who spend too much time alone:

1. The concept of *communio* to further articulate what it is we seek in our relationships

2. The histories and characteristics of the 'righteous Gentiles,' to discover with whom we might be able to cultivate communio

I present this material, not to stitch up a theory of community development, but, rather, as angles that might be used fruitfully in our efforts. For example, I am not dealing with the structures in civil society most conducive to the nurture of communio. Based on my own experience as a community development worker, I find myself agreeing with John Reader (1994), who argues that so often "those who set out to create community seem doomed to disappointment." Reader proposes that the concept and experience of communio as meaningful, valued togetherness can open up new pathways towards the goal of building community (1994, pp. 60-61).

Communio can become a vision of universal human solidarity, which can reconcile closeness and distance.[9] Communio is: verb rather than noun; praxis rather than goal; activity rather than product; participation rather than membership; embarking rather than arriving; fickle rather than fixed; insecure rather than stitched up; adventure rather than feat; desire and disappointment, rather than destination. David L. Fleming (1997) explains that communio is the Latin equivalent of the Greek word *koinonia*. He goes on to say:

> In Latin we may make a distinction between the words communio and communitas, which underlines the emphasis we are trying to grasp. Communitas is a word to apply to a certain objective or substantive reality . . . a group of people who are together, having something in common. Communio, for its part, emphasizes the process or the actual sharing and thus the dynamism or energy necessary for a community to become and to remain a community. (p. 1)

If we are talking about the energy that initiates, fuses and maintains social relationships beyond the family, rather than a highly contested apparently static state called community, then how can we set about releasing and nurturing that energy? The shift of focus from a "substantive reality" to a process–a process that binds people in friendship and comradeship–implies a shift away from concentrating solely on developing structures and organizations to a process which allows people to come to know each other personally. The 'social capital' theorists have identified bonding, linking and bridging relationships as constitutive of social capital–a quality created between people, often described as glue, trust, mutuality, and respect. We can see these relationships very simply as:[10]

- bonding–with family, close friends, and a close network
- linking–to institutions, business, government

- bridging–to a wider network, or networks, within the community, immediate reference or support group (Hampshire, 2000)

Many of us benefit from bonded relationships characterized by a blend of acceptance, challenge, mutuality and imbalance, conformity and its companion of threatened rejection, honesty, duty, tradition, constraint, and freedom. In Australia, people with disability benefit greatly from the commitment of their families. Beyond the walls of institutionalized care, this is the realm of social life in which people with impairments are most likely to carry out their lives. Conversely, we also know that many people 'living in the community' only ever see paid workers and do not have family, workmates, friends or comrades.

Establishing solidarity away from home, on that "farther shore," can be encouraged by social networks that help translate an 'I' mentality into a 'we' mentality. The concept of communio speaks to the possibilities for bridging relationships. The dilemma here is that people come to know each other personally and, thence, to enjoy communio–which must surely contribute to breaking down loneliness and rejection–as a consequence of other activities. Reader (1994) suggests, then, that "we need to know under what circumstances it is possible for people to meet and work together in this informal manner" (p. 61). Notice his use of the term *work*. Groups that are capable of offering the life-giving acceptance and solidarity that so many people with disability yearn for do not emerge as lifestyle fun clubs. They require a "common cause and motivation, as well as time and space" (Reader, 1994, p. 61). He goes on to assert that "recent changes in social life are making the latter two increasingly difficult to find" (p. 61). Common cause and motivation are also extremely problematic in this area of our work of embrace.

We are inviting people into the lives of stigmatized people who are considered burdensome, disturbing, frightening, incapable of mutuality, demanding, or just plain unworthy and less than human. Many people with impairments are seen as the irremediably troubling *other*. We know that just being in a place or hoping for a friend to emerge do not overcome deeply ingrained practices of exclusion. I do not believe that participation in active, working social networks is a form of therapy that will fix people up; neither do I think that strengthening bridging relationships in the lives of people with disability will substantially undermine the social mechanisms that construct disability and impose a devalued social status on them. No amount of wishful thinking and talk on our part will change the reality of those stigmas and the fears they engender in resistant others. But it is possible (though not assured) that communio will emerge when people can breach that initial estrangement. So, the question remains, is there any way into people's hearts?

Do we have any historical resources that show individuals stepping into the breach and forging powerful connections with people who are socially reviled? Clearly, there are those amongst us–citizen advocates, neighbors, chaplains, friends, and comrades–pursuing and enjoying creative, constructive, occasionally protective, relationships with previously disparaged persons, sometimes within organizations and sometimes within informal social networks.[11] Looking at who enters these relationships and why can give us further insights into the processes that bind people to each other. I think that recent studies into the activities and characteristics of 'the righteous Gentiles'–the people who altruistically responded to the Jews in Europe during the 1930s and 1940s–reveal many hope-giving possibilities.[12] One of those people was a Polish man, Jan Karski, who says:

> The Jews were abandoned by governments, by church hierarchies, by existing societal structures. But they were not abandoned by all of humanity. . . . There were thousands upon thousands of people in Europe who risked their life for the Jews. They were priests, nuns, workers, peasants, enlightened ones, simpletons–from all walks of life. They were good people, very simply. We have more good people than probably we think we have in humanity.[13]

Surely we can say that, at a time when we know people with disability to be abandoned by many, all of humanity has not walked away. Who were, and are, these good people (estimated to number 100,000; 11,000 of whom have been honored)? David Gushee (1994) reports that in his prolonged research he has asked these questions of rescuers–a cross-section of European society at the time. He says:

> Rescuers were men and women from every nation in Nazi-dominated Europe. They were rich and poor, young and old, people from all social classes and occupations. When politically affiliated, rescuers tended to be involved more with democratic and leftist groups than with rightist parties, but they could be found all across the political spectrum. . . . Rescuers are more likely to have been people with a strong sense of social responsibility, and capacity to empathize with suffering people. They also tend to demonstrate a consistent commitment to helping needy people, before and after the Holocaust as well as during it. Rescuers tended to be people with a healthy self-esteem and a sense of independence and competence. . . . Some rescuers appear to have been adventuresome types, and others drew upon a sense of social marginality as a resource for compassion. Another mark of rescuer character is the nearly universal unwillingness to accept praise for their deeds. "It is what anyone would have done," they say of behavior that almost no-one did. For

them, to rescue Jews was the perfectly natural and obvious course of action. People needed help, so help was offered. (Gushee, 1994, p. 32)

This is a social profile of people who, when asked what motivated them, spoke of: personal ties with Jews, group influence, patriotic or political convictions, a commitment to justice, human rights, care and compassion, moral obligation to care, religious–especially Christian–convictions, and some were unable to give a clear reason "beyond the fact that they were simply moved to the depths of their being by the plight of a Jewish person or family desperately in trouble" (Gushee, 1994, p. 35). This is what Erik Erikson has called the opposite of *rejectivity*. It is born from *shakenness*: the state experienced by those who have seen through the dominant lie that some amongst us must be excluded or exterminated for our protection. Jan Patoka, a Czech philosopher and martyr of the 1900s, saw this shakenness as pivotal in the move from fearing our fellows to embracing them.[14]

Gushee's conclusions are echoed in many studies about rescuers. Whilst it is potentially misleading to use the term 'rescuer' in any discussion about disability, these profiles reveal the capacity of people in all places and situations to react without fear in the face of pain, and to create spaces in their lives for others; indeed, to affirm the future of the abandoned person. I do not pretend that talk of the rescuers undoes the horror of the Shoah; I do not wish to detract from the vitality of the memories of the victims. I do not imagine that talking of righteousness in this way will bring an end to all contemporary attacks upon the socially undesirable, wherever or whoever they are.

However, I believe that a reachable "farther shore" is not so much a place to attain as a journey to be made in company. I believe that learning about people who did not raise their arm to repel Jews and reviled others but extended their hands in solidarity reminds us that the sum of humanity is not somehow naturally resistant to those with impairments. We also have some idea about those whom we should be searching out in the hope that communio can enrich our corporate lives. We know that we should not be afraid of asking hard actions of people. We know that righteousness is not the preserve of an elite but the genuine uprising of all types of people. And we know the sorts of traits we can encourage to take root in our hearts.

These conclusions open up many possibilities for the simple yet extremely difficult significance of risking care (another over-worn word, but nonetheless important to stress in a world that says of disability, cure it or kill it). Communio flowering amongst the righteous and those who would engage all people in the demands of daily loving is the opposite of rejectivity. In its shakenness, it proclaims truth to the powerful lies of the Coca-Cola community and all its shady companions. Yes, Heaney's hope remains alive. "A farther shore is reachable from here"–a shore on the far side of revenge, regret, suspicion, and rejection. And it is a shore at our door.

NOTES

1. Although, I find myself wanting to imagine a non-repentant prodigal daughter whose sheer defiance and survival skills make the gracious father rethink his approach to forgiveness (and where is the mother anyway?), or someone talking of the dangers of teaching young children that those they have daily physical contact with are a source of infection rather than fun!

2. I am confirmed in this after hearing a scientist asserting that Australians are reluctant to give him and his colleagues the go-ahead on human cloning because we have not had enough community education on its benefits. Now, I consider that my apprehensions about human cloning are grounded not in ignorance but in real ethical concerns. No amount of community education about the wonders of this sort of science will induce me to see that ethical questions have no place in deciding where resources are put, and, indeed, how we interact with the rudiments of human existence. So, if I feel like this, isn't it possible that the resistances others have to social-change strategies are also unlikely to yield to education aimed at correcting their ignorance. Perhaps the failure to welcome people with disability is more about other fears or the need to find scapegoats than it is about ignorance.

3. Gertrude MacIntyre (1997), Active partners: Education and community development, *International Journal of Social Economics*, vol. 24, no. 11, p. 1290 ff. (Electronic version: Expanded Academic, p. 10 of 12 pages).

4. Gertrude MacIntyre (1997) goes on to state: "If you look back in history, the concept of community has emerged as an old order declined and a new one emerged. Saint Augustine wrote *The City of God* when barbarians besieged Rome. Monasteries developed as the Roman Empire declined and Europe plunged into darkness. Sir Thomas Moore wrote *Utopia* in 1516 as Henry VIII extended his power and set about privatizing the monasteries and the wealthy extended their holdings at the expense of the poor" (MacIntyre, 1997, p. 1 [Electronic version]).

5. I recently saw this sort of community described as "a lifestyle enclave." How might we describe the lifestyle enclave of homeless people?

6. Dietrich Bonhoeffer (1932): "Freedom is not a quality of a person, nor is it an ability, capacity, or attribute . . . Freedom is not a possession, a thing, or an object. Freedom is a relationship, indeed, between two persons." (in *Creation and Fall: A Theological Interpretation of Genesis 1-3*, republished in 1959, New York: Macmillan).

7. It can be argued that, in the context of immigration, "familiarity" is "the staunchest enemy of inquisitiveness and criticism" for sociological thinking (Bauman, 1990, p. 15). Confronted with this common-sense familiarity, which constantly reasserts the given and unquestioned assumptions in the field, the task of sociology as it is defined by Bauman is to act "as a meddlesome and often irritating stranger" [cited in N. Albertsen and B. Diken (2000), Introduction: Immigrants on the Margin (draft), retrieved from: http://www.comp.lancaster.ac.uk/sociology/soc038bd.html]

8. Electronic version: Expanded Academic.

9. For more information and ideas about the development of this idea, which emerges from traditional views of community, read Robert Gascoigne, *The public forum and Christian ethics*, Cambridge: Cambridge University Press, 2000.

10. Robert Putnam, describer of past community (and hence a not entirely believable romantic), documenter of current community decay, and dreamer after an American society in which people no longer bowl alone, is the acknowledged progenitor of social capital theory. Read R. Putman, *Bowling alone: The collapse and revival of American community*, New York: Simon and Schuster, 2000, to explore his ideas further.

11. I promised to keep the skeptical side of the dialectic going; so, if you are interested in the sheer malevolence of the apparently altruistic, read Toni Morrison's *The Bluest Eye*, Chatto and Windus: London, 1979. Her description of the social worker is chilling.

12. I use the term 'righteous Gentiles' as it is the official title given by Yad Vashem, of the Holocaust Center, to describe the non-Jewish rescuers of Jews during the Shoah. I recognize, though, that there is debate amongst Jewish scholars about the appropriateness of the term. For example, Berel Lang (1997, p. 91), in her article, "For and Against the 'Righteous Gentiles'" (non-Jewish defenders of Jewish lives during the Holocaust), seeks to describe these people as heroes, and thence to restore righteousness to those many people who, in smaller ways, refused to cooperate with the Nazis or to profit from the murder of Jews. He concludes: "To identify and honor those who are heroic means that the burden of being 'righteous' goes back where it belongs, in the day-to-day life of ordinary people who are not and perhaps cannot be heroes, but who are nonetheless responsible for knowing and acting on the principles of common humanity. That is, for being righteous" (p. 6).

13. Jan Karski, a 'righteous Gentile,' quoted in Eva Fogelman, Rescuers of Jews During the Holocaust: A Model for a Caring Community, retrieved June 1995, from Schindler's List Teaching Guide: http://dept.english.upenn.edu/~afilreis/Holocaust/rescuers_article.html. Fogelman is also author of *Conscience and Courage: Rescuers of Jews during the Holocaust*. The book, in Fogelman's words, "traces the psychological making of a rescuer." She says: "I began, after a while, to wait for the recital of one or more of those well known passages: a nurturing, loving home: an altruistic parent or beloved caretaker who served as a role model for altruistic behavior; a tolerance for people who were different; a childhood illness or personal loss that tested their resilience and exposed them to special care; and an upbringing that emphasized independence, discipline, with explanations, rather than physical punishment or withdrawal of love, and caring" (ibid.).

14. For further exploration of the connection between shakenness and social movement activity, see A. Shanks' (2000) *God and Modernity: A New Way to Do Theology*.

REFERENCES

Bauman, Z. (1990). *Thinking sociologically*. Oxford: Blackwell.

Bonhoeffer, D. (1932). *Creation and fall: A theological interpretation of Genesis 1-3* (republished 1959). New York: Macmillan.

Buber, M. (1958). *I and thou*. Edinburgh: T. T. Clark.

Fleming, D. L. (1997). Communion: Divine life enlarging our desires. *Review for Religious*, March-April. First presented as a part of the Symposium on Community and Consecrated Life, held at the Jesuit Center for Spiritual Growth, Wernersville, Pennsylvania, in October 1996. Retrieved July 7, 2003, from: http://www.review forreligious.org/indices/1990.html

Fogelman, E. Rescuers of Jews during the Holocaust: A model for a caring community. Retrieved from: http://dept.english.upenn.edu/~afilreis/Holocaust/rescuers_article.html

Fogelman, E. (1997). *Conscience and courage: Rescuers of Jews during the Holocaust.* New York: Doubleday.

Fries, K. (1997). *Staring back: Disability experience from the inside out.* New York: Plume.

Gasgoigne, R. (2000). *The public forum and Christian ethics.* Cambridge: Cambridge University Press.

Gushee, D. P. (1994). Why they helped the Jews: What we can learn from the righteous Gentiles of the Holocaust. *Christianity Today, vol. 38*, no. 12, p. 32 (4). Hampshire, A. (2000). Stronger communities and social connectedness: Social capital in practice. Executive Strategy Unit, The Benevolent Society (Paddington, NSW) presented to *The Council on the Ageing National Congress*, in November 2000.

Jeffers, F. E. (1996). Love and the relatedness of things. *The Humanist, vol. 56*, no. 1, Jan-Feb, p. 21 (2).

Lang, B. (1997). For and against the "righteous Gentiles." *Mark Judaism: A Quarterly Journal of Jewish Life and Thought, vol. 46*, no. 1, Winter.

MacIntyre, G. (1997). Active partners: Education and community development. *International Journal of Social Economics, vol. 24*, no. 11, p. 1290 ff. (Electronic version).

Morrison, T. (1979). *The bluest eye.* London: Chatto and Windus.

Putnam, R. (2000). *Bowling alone: The collapse and revival of American community.* New York: Simon & Schuster.

Reader, J. (1994). *Local theology: Church and community in dialogue.* London: SPCK.

Shanks, A. (2000). God and modernity: A new and better way to do theology. London: Routledge.

The Buddhist Insight of Emptiness as an Antidote for the Model of Deficient Humanness Contained Within the Label 'Intellectually Disabled'

Peter W. Hawkins, BA, MA

SUMMARY. There is, in Buddhism, a teaching called *sunyata*, or emptiness. This teaching is tersely presented in a Mahayana text referred to as "The Heart Sutra." The theme of this sutra is that all phenomena are empty of separate being, and this is the basis of resolving all apparent dualisms: in this case, referring to *intellectually disabled* and *not intellectually disabled*. Put posi-

---

Peter W. Hawkins, spent twelve years, from 1990 to 2002, working in the field of support for people with intellectual disabilities, and for the last four worked as an advocate with Independent Advocacy SA Inc. Between the time of writing this article, and its publication, he has become a Buddhist monk, now known as Thich Truc Thong Phap.

Address correspondence to: Peter Hawkins, c/o Craig Hawkins, 35 Bombay Street, Oaklands, 5046, South Australia, Australia.

This paper is dedicated to the memory of Efstathios (Stephen) Tettis (9 July 1957-10 July 2001), a patient teacher who is alive in the work I do.

The article is based on a paper presented by Peter W. Hawkins at the Third National Conference on Spirituality and Disability, held in Melbourne in October, 2001: Peter Hawkins (2002), in C. Newell (Ed.), *Exclusion and embrace: Conversations about spirituality and disability.* Melbourne: UnitingCare, 2002.

[Haworth co-indexing entry note]: "The Buddhist Insight of Emptiness as an Antidote for the Model of Deficient Humanness Contained Within the Label 'Intellectually Disabled.'" Hawkins, Peter W. Co-published simultaneously in *Journal of Religion, Disability & Health* (The Haworth Pastoral Press, an imprint of The Haworth Press, Inc.) Vol. 8, No. 1/2, 2004, pp. 45-54; and: *Voices in Disability and Spirituality from the Land Down Under: Outback to Outfront* (ed: Christopher Newell, and Andy Calder) The Haworth Pastoral Press, an imprint of The Haworth Press, Inc., 2004, pp. 45-54. Single or multiple copies of this article are available for a fee from The Haworth Document Delivery Service [1-800-HAWORTH, 9:00 a.m. - 5:00 p.m. (EST). E-mail address: docdelivery@haworthpress.com].

Digital Object Identifier: 10.1300/J095v8n01_05

tively, it is called *interbeing*, and it critiques hierarchical notions that derive from dualistic notions. This critique is explicated clearly within the context of an open and loving relationship between a person labeled 'intellectually disabled' and another person, the author, who does not have that label and who moves from being a support worker in the man's life to being a lifelong friend. *[Article copies available for a fee from The Haworth Document Delivery Service: 1-800-HAWORTH. E-mail address: <docdelivery@haworthpress.com> Website: <http://www.HaworthPress.com> © 2004 by The Haworth Press, Inc. All rights reserved.]*

KEYWORDS. Intellectual disability, religion, Buddhism, interbeing

THE HEART OF THE PRAJÑAPARAMITA

The Bodhisattva Avalokita, while moving in the deep course of Perfect Understanding, shed light on the five skandhas and found them equally empty. After this penetration, he overcame all pain.

Listen, Shariputra, form is emptiness, emptiness is form, form does not differ from emptiness, and emptiness does not differ from form. The same is true with feelings, perceptions, mental formations, and consciousness.

Hear, Shariputra, all dharmas are marked with emptiness; they are neither produced nor destroyed, neither defiled nor immaculate, neither increasing, nor decreasing. Therefore, in emptiness there is neither form, nor feeling, nor tongue, or body, or mind, no form, no sound, no smell, no taste, no touch, no object of mind; no realms of elements (from eyes to mind consciousness); no interdependent origins and no extinction of them (from ignorance to old age and death): no suffering, no origination of suffering, no extinction of suffering, no path; no understanding, no attainment.

Because there is no attainment, the bodhisattvas, supported by the Perfection of Understanding, find no obstacles for their minds. Having no obstacles, they overcome fear, liberating themselves forever from illusion and realising perfect Nirvana. All Buddhas in the past, present, and future, thanks to this Perfect Understanding, arrive at full, right, and universal Enlightenment.

Therefore, one should know that Perfect Understanding is a great mantra, is the highest mantra, is the unequalled mantra, the destroyer of all suffering, the incorruptible truth. A mantra of Prajñaparamita should therefore be proclaimed. This is the mantra:

Gate gate paragate parasamgate bodhi svaha.

INTRODUCTION

This *sutra* is a well-known scripture in the Mahayana tradition of Buddhism, and is recited daily in Zen monasteries. By way of introducing it to you, I would like to invite you to engage in a short reflection about the actual sheet of paper you are reading. This contemplation is based on one composed by the Venerable Thich Nhat Hanh, a Vietnamese Zen master who is the author of the commentary on the Heart Sutra which I refer to in this paper.

As you look at this piece of paper and use your imagination, you may be able to see a cloud floating in it. Without a cloud, there is no rain; without rain, there are no trees; and without trees, this paper would not exist. The cloud is essential to the existence of the paper: if there is no cloud, there can be no sheet of paper. The word coined by Thich Nhat Hanh to name this relationship is *interbeing*. The cloud and the paper *inter-are*.

This is true of sunshine and the paper too. Without the sunshine, the paper cannot exist, because the forest from which the trees are taken would not be able to grow. Looking more deeply, we can see the forestry worker who felled the tree and took it to the mill to transform it into paper. Then there is the wheat that had to be farmed to produce the food for the forestry worker. And then there are all of the ancestors of the forestry worker in the paper as well.

We are in the paper too, because when we look at the paper, it is part of our perception. Our mind is also part of this paper. Everything inter-is with the paper: time, space and all the phenomena that have made up the history of the universe, including the human mind. This sheet of paper does not exist by itself alone; it exists because everything else exists.

If we were to remove one of the elements that make up the paper, such as the sunshine, it could not exist. Nothing exists separately from anything else. Everything that is, the logger, the cloud, the sunshine and so on, provides the occasion for everything else to exist. Everything holds everything in being. There is no separately existing entity while this paper contains non-paper elements without which it cannot exist. What, then, is meant in the sutra, by emptiness?

I love the first verse of the Heart Sutra. I imagine Avalokita as a deep-sea fish moving slowly over the ocean floor, fully aware, whilst searching for nutriment. Avalokita came to his "Perfect Understanding" not simply intellectually but with his whole being, and it transformed his whole being to the extent that "he overcame all pain." And what did he come to understand? He understood that the human being, made up of both physical and mental factors, is, at the ultimate level, empty of separate being. Our notion of a distinct, permanent and self-existent *Me* as opposed to *You* is false, and all of our consequent identifications are ultimately false. This wrong view is understood to be the cause of all confusion and pain in the world, and is so because it is the basis of dualistic thinking, which results in polarities of *self* over and against *other*.

Some other dualities which drive our way of relating to the world include mind/spirit versus flesh, male versus female, human versus non-human, dark versus light, disabled versus whole, and sane versus insane. These dualities are manifest in many of the destructive systems that we have come to know as sexism, classism, racism, and so forth. Perhaps the most frightening of the consequences of dualism is that we have set ourselves over and against the very planet of which we are a part. If we refer to our reflective meditation, we realize that, in Buddhist terms, we exist as a result of a constellation of ever-changing and interactive conditions. There is no chicken and egg argument possible in this understanding, for both arise in relation to each other.

There are, in this teaching, no discrete entities in the world: nothing is separable from, or remains untouched by, whatever else exists in relation to it. Everything in the universe is held in being by everything else in the universe, and all things (or *dharmas*) are conditioned in relation to each other. This teaching is the Buddhist Genesis statement. One of the earliest formulations of this teaching is contained within the following terse statement: this being, that becomes; from the arising of this, that arises; this not being, that becomes not; from the ceasing of this, that ceases.

What is really real about the universe, in terms of the Heart Sutra, is that everything, all dharmas including us, is irrevocably part of a web of inter-existence. In reality, no greater value can be ascribed to one dharma than to another. The problem is with the way the human mind works, wrongly perceiving dharmas as separate, discrete, permanent, and either something I want or something I don't want. Avalokita understood with his whole being that, in reality, all dharmas are marked with emptiness; they are neither produced nor destroyed, neither increasing nor decreasing, neither defiled nor immaculate, neither disabled (read culturally devalued) nor fully valued.

MEETING MY TEACHER

In February 1990 I got a job with a respite and recreational program in Adelaide, called Stepping Out. I was to go out with a man called Stephen

Tettis for three hours on a Sunday. I was told that he would be fairly resistant and that I would probably have to chase him around the dining room table to catch him in order to dress him. On the first Sunday, I arrived at his family home with a Disability Services Officer (DSO) from Strathmont Centre, who was going to come out with us the first time round. We did get Stephen dressed, really with the minimum of fuss, and then went to Balaklava to watch a football match. The DSO sat in the back, and seemed to me to be one of those workers who have become as institutionalized as the Strathmont residents. I felt a little uneasy about talking to Stephen with him there, in case he might think that I thought Stephen was a real person; nevertheless, I talked with Stephen a little. At one point later in the afternoon, I was startled by Stephen's hand reaching across to me, waiting to be shaken. So I took his lovely warm hand and shook it. The next week, and forever after, when I arrived he would be standing at the front gate, fully clothed and with a water bottle, waiting for his new buddy.

In 1990 the Western and Orthodox Churches had Easter at the same time. This was a month or so after Stephen and I started spending time together. So, on our mutual Easter Day, I picked him up as usual and off we drove to Strathalbyn with a pile of Easter eggs for a friend of mine who lives on a small farm. It was a beautiful day and we listened to lots of music on the way. On the road I had been thinking that what separated Stephen, an Orthodox Christian, and myself, at that time a candidate for ordination in the Anglican Church, was the interpretation of the *filioque* clause in the Nicene Creed. This clause is concerned with the dynamics of the relationship between God the Son and God the Holy Spirit in relation to God the Father within the broader Catholic teaching concerning the Holy Trinity. I then wondered if being a Christian was to do with our capacity to subscribe to certain theological propositions. If that were so, how could Stephen, whose capacity to understand the highly conceptualized field of Christian theology was probably not well developed, be a Christian?

As we pulled into my friend's drive, and these thoughts were coming to an end, again Stephen reached across to me and, as if on cue, took my hand to shake it and smiled beautifully at me with his eyes full of love-light. All my concerns about his Christianity were instantly put to rest and, from that time, my sense of who he was, my love and respect for him, and my commitment to him grew exponentially.

Stephen would never get out of the car to go into a café or to visit someone's house; we had to bring the coffee out to him, open his car door and sit around him. One day I decided to take him to Murray Bridge to visit my sister and her family, who were very open to people labeled intellectually disabled. From experience, I knew that Stephen would get out of the car, go to the front door, and run away as soon as somebody answered it. I rang my sister first to ask if she and her family would leave the front door open, let us come in and sit in the sitting room, and then they could quietly come in and gather around us. This strategy worked, and very soon after this, when Stephen realized he was perfectly safe to venture out with me, we started to go into shops, cafés, homes, and public transport.

Many possibilities that could enrich his life began to open up to him. We would often catch the tram to Glenelg, which he loved to do. We caught the Steam Ranger from Adelaide to Victor Harbour and picnicked on the delicious Greek food his mother had prepared for us. I established the goal of going on a camp, and in our third year together we went on a family camp where he did things we never thought possible, including staying away from home at night–and sleeping.

There were many experiences to be had that deepened my understanding of his vulnerabilities, his competencies, and my preparedness to advocate for him. What developed was a mutual love that sustained us right up until his death in July 2001. Another aspect of this was the relationship that developed between myself and his family, his mother, his sisters, his niece and nephew, and his extended family. These relationships sustained me and nurtured my openness to and love of him. His family saw that this was possible; that there were people in the world who also cared deeply for Stephen and could be trusted with him.

THE TEACHINGS AND THE TEACHER

How do these two things fit together? To my mind, the relationship that grew over eleven years and will remain important to me all of my days is a clear indication of interbeing. Stephen's life and being were some of the conditions that provided for the growth of my understanding and commitment, and have led to my work as an advocate–quite apart from everything else that I can only be because of him. Who I was to him and because of him meant that he had access to very conscious and committed support, which opened up possibilities of experience in his life, that had not existed prior to my presence in it.

I am not a self that is separate from Stephen: who I am contains many elements that come about as a result of the relationship. He was not a self that was separate from me: who he was contained many elements that come about as a result of the relationship. I am who I am and he was who he was because of the relationship we had.

What Does This Mean in Terms of the Deficiency-Based Model of Humanness Contained in the Term 'Intellectual Disability'?

Early in the relationship with Stephen, there were people who would say to me, "He'd be better taken." This was said in spite of the fact that he was leading a very rich life of family, work, and recreational commitments. Once, on a bus, a lady hissed, "It shouldn't be allowed." This came out of the fact that Stephen, who engaged in a number of self-stimulating behaviors, was vocalizing loudly and gesticulating with his hands. After he had died someone said to me, "He's better off dead." "No," I answered, "he's better off dancing his way down Wakefield Street to the Glenelg tram, or eating his way through a scone with jam and cream."

Death is what we foist on those whom we see as other in relation to ourselves and judge as lesser than ourselves. This death wish can express itself in many ways. For Stephen, I believe it was expressed in a lack of good health advocacy on the part of the health professionals who dealt with him over the last two years of his life. It was also expressed, in terms of the impact it had on his life, in being sacked from his sheltered workshop when his productive capacity fell short of the demands made by the intrusion of economic rationalism into the sheltered workshop system.

More generally, this death wish is expressed in the lack of government funding, and imagination, to provide options for people with additional support needs; including accommodation, inclusive education, meaningful, and properly remunerated work, real involvement in community, and the right to have and keep their children.

Recently I saw the death wish expressed in a Web site that belongs to an extreme eugenics organization called the Prometheist Church. One of the principles and goals of the Prometheists, a North-American-based organization, is "to create a genetically enhanced race that will eventually become a new, superior species. In the short term, this will be achieved via eugenics and genetic engineering." Further, they say:

> Potential children are in abundant supply and the world is overpopulated with people without a future. Every child brought into this world should be of the finest intellect possible, and free of genetic diseases or abnormalities. Every generation needs to be an incremental step in the evolution to a new species.

I joined a chat board advertised on the Prometheist website and posed the following question (the details of which are perfectly true):

One of the reasons I have joined this group is to discover what people involved in eugenics generally, and interested in what one might call 'an upward evolutionary trend,' think about what we in Australia call 'intellectual disability' and what, I think, people in the USA call 'mental retardation.' I have a dear cousin who has Down's syndrome, and it bothers me that she might not have a place in the world envisioned by Prometheists. Perhaps you could allay my fears or provide me with some clear thinking about how you see such people in your vision of humanity's future. While I am certainly in favor of an upward trend in an evolutionary sense, I would miss my cousin if she were not in that world with me. I look forward to hearing people's views on this.

I received a few answers; the most extreme response, which another respondent agreed with, was as follows:

Retards are non-viable humans placed in the correct classification of Freaks or Monsters. Anyone who raises a retard is wasting their time, and one would have to doubt the intelligence of the person devoting 20+ years of time to such a freak/monster. Why bother raising a creature like that when one could just as easily look after a normal viable human instead? Ones [sic] best option is to terminate all creatures of that extreme degenerate nature at the soonest possible time. Bottom line: Retards are a total waste of time and resources not only on the parents but on society as a whole. In my book such an action as raising/protecting retards would be a sin/crime.

Dr. Wolf Wolfensberger (1987) offers a very comprehensive discussion of 'deathmaking' in his monograph, *The New Genocide of Handicapped and Afflicted People*. He draws the reader's attention to the human tendency to create identities and dualities, through which certain people are devalued and seen as dangerous, non-human or sub-human, worthless, and a drain on community resources. While dualism devalues some, such as Stephen Tettis, it places a higher value on others such as myself. This duality contains the extremes of defiled and immaculate, referred to in the Heart Sutra. Wolfensberger points out that at times of social stress, rather than thinking through the true causes of the stressful conditions and solving them at the base, the vulnerable *other* is scapegoated, and in extreme circumstances, such as during the Third Reich, such people are murdered (1987, pp. 7-8). Further, Professor Wolfensberger defines 'deathmaking' as "any actions or patterns of actions which either directly or indirectly bring about or hasten the death of a person or group" (1987, p. 1).

The Buddhist understanding that I have considered in this paper would summarize these typical cultural misperceptions in the following three ways:

- We are discrete selves encased by rigid identifications, like 'disabled' or 'non-disabled,' and are subject to fear, hatred, greed and confusion.
- We are not interdependent phenomena who help each other happen by providing the context or conditions for our unfolding.
- We ascribe value to the other and ourselves which is hierarchical, dangerous, and does not take into account that which is really real.

The teaching of the Heart Sutra strikes at the core of these very dangerous misperceptions, and allows for interbeing which, in the Buddhist experience, gives rise to understanding, acceptance, generosity, a joy in each other's being, and inclusiveness. The teaching provides an explanation of what our wrong view is based on, while a deep spiritual practice reconditions our minds and hearts, and enables us to see things as they really are. To this extent, the Heart Sutra critiques the notion of disability, whose offspring are exclusion, abandonment, and death.

THE TEACHER PASSES AWAY

After eighteen months of slowly wasting away, with neither successful medical intervention nor any real attempt at intervention (at least, in my view), Steven was admitted to the Wakefield Hospital for the last time. It was a Tuesday evening when his sister rang me and I went down to the hospital. The nurses gave him little hope of seeing the night out. They came in about 10.30 PM to turn him in bed; it was very traumatic for him: he groaned and shook in fear and pain. I knelt by his bed and gently stroked the palm of that big hand which had reached out to me eleven years before, on our first day together.

He grasped my hand and stared straight into my eyes. I knelt there, holding his hands and praying that he would know he was not alone. Slowly he calmed down and went to sleep. I went home at one o'clock. The next Monday I called in to see him for his forty-fourth birthday. He lay very still, breathing very lightly; I sat and watched for a while. The next morning his sister rang me to tell me that he had passed away. I arrived as the undertaker was removing him in his body bag. His sister insisted that they open the body bag so that I might see him. His funeral was held later that week. Approximately two hundred people came to the church.

My teacher had passed away. Without him, eleven years of learning and growth would not have been possible. But the gift I treasure most was the trust he invested in me. This trust enabled him to rest easy, look deeply into my face, and overcome the fear and pain that he encountered in the simple experience of being turned in the bed. The interbeing nature of our relationship was manifest right through to the end of his life, and I shall never forget it.

REFERENCE

Wolfensberger, W. (1987). *The new genocide of handicapped and afflicted people* (2nd revised edition). Syracuse, NY: Syracuse University Training Group.

Judaism, Spirituality, and Disability: An Australian Perspective

Melinda Jones, BA, LLB

SUMMARY. Judaism teaches that the wisdom to resolve current issues can be found in ancient texts. While there are many references in the written and oral law pertaining to disability, these are not well known and, being taken out of context, are at risk of misinterpretation. This article draws on *Halacha*, the ancient Jewish law which literally means "the way on which one goes," to demonstrate that the principles of Judaism and rules for daily living have the potential to empower people with disabilities. It argues that Jewish spirituality involves the recognition of the role of Hashem in the way we live our lives and involves adherence to ethical standards, the most important of which is "choose life." Because all lives are of infinite value, all must be treated with dignity and respect. Yet Judaism as practiced in Australia and elsewhere has often excluded people with disabilities or simply ignored our need for inclusion. *[Article copies available for a fee from The Haworth Document Delivery Service: 1-800-HAWORTH. E-mail address: <docdelivery@haworthpress.com> Website: <http://www.HaworthPress.com> © 2004 by The Haworth Press, Inc. All rights reserved.]*

Melinda Jones is a human rights scholar and activist, a feminist legal theorist, a person with a disability, a traditional Orthodox Jew, and the mother of 5 children. She is the former Director of the Australian Human Rights Centre and former Senior Lecture in Law at UNSW.

Address correspondence to: Melinda Jones, Faculty of Law, University of NSW, Sydney, NSW 2052, Australia (E-mail: m.jones@unsw.edu.au).

[Haworth co-indexing entry note]: "Judaism, Spirituality, and Disability: An Australian Perspective." Jones, Melinda. Co-published simultaneously in *Journal of Religion, Disability & Health* (The Haworth Pastoral Press, an imprint of The Haworth Press, Inc.) Vol. 8, No. 1/2, 2004, pp. 55-88; and: *Voices in Disability and Spirituality from the Land Down Under: Outback to Outfront* (ed: Christopher Newell, and Andy Calder) The Haworth Pastoral Press, an imprint of The Haworth Press, Inc., 2004, pp. 55-88. Single or multiple copies of this article are available for a fee from The Haworth Document Delivery Service [1-800-HAWORTH, 9:00 a.m. - 5:00 p.m. (EST). E-mail address: docdelivery@haworthpress.com].

KEYWORDS. Judaism, Jewish law, disability, religion, spirituality

In the ancient Jewish text, the B'raita, Rabbi Yossi is recorded as saying:

> Once I was walking in the darkness and I saw a blind man who was walking with a torch in his hand. I asked him, "My son, why do you need this torch?" He told me, "As long as this torch is in my hand people can see me and save me from thorns and ditches." (Talmud Bavli, Megillah 24b)

A significant aspect of disability is the failure of the community to see and respond to the difficulties confronting people with disabilities. This passage suggests, however, that once a torch is lit and the individual is made visible, those in the broader community will take responsibility for removing obstacles that interfere with the full participation of people with disabilities.

The range of experiences included in the category of 'disability,' and the types of barriers confronted by people with disabilities, is broad. *Disability* includes physical disabilities (such as mobility impairment), intellectual disabilities (referred to as 'mental disabilities' in the US), sensory disabilities (vision, hearing and speech impairments), psychiatric disabilities (including the full range of so-called mental illnesses), and chronic illness. While, historically, disabilities have been seen as limitations resulting from the medical or pathological state of the 'disabled individual,' today the limitations experienced by people with disabilities are seen to be context-specific–to the extent that what is *disabling* in one environment may be *enabling* in another. Just as the ability of the blind man mentioned above depended not just on his visual impairment but also on the willingness of others to remove barriers and to make the environment friendly, it is now accepted by people with disabilities, activists and scholars that much that is disabling is socially constructed.[1]

In modern industrialized societies such as Australia, people with disabilities have been, until very recently, both out of sight and out of mind. Most people with disabilities, including Jews with disabilities, have been hidden away, segregated from the mainstream of society, sent to different schools than their brothers and sisters, and/or sent to live out their days in institutions. In the exclusionary process, the very existence of people with disabilities has been privatized, relegated to the realm of domestic and family affairs. Being Jewish does not exempt people with disabilities from the attitudes and treatments generally accepted in the society in which they live as legitimate ways of dealing with people with disabilities.

Issues for people with disabilities in Australia are similar to those of people with disabilities all around the world. For example, people with disabilities are often seen as abnormal, aberrant, strange, ugly disfigured things that should be kept away from ordinary people.[2] Further, people with disabilities have been the objects of scorn and hatred, and are rarely treated with the dignity and respect to which they are entitled.[3] They have been placed in institutions where they have been starved, subjected to cruel and inhuman treatment, locked in small rooms, denied any stimulus and hidden from the wider community.[4] In Australia, as elsewhere, a high percentage of women with intellectual disabilities have been involuntarily sterilized for reasons of eugenics or because of the fear of pregnancy from widespread sexual assault.[5] What's more, children have been segregated and schooled in inferior 'special schools,' even though significant research has been undertaken which has shown that excluding children from the ordinary school system is harmful to all concerned and cannot even be defended on economic grounds.[6] Beyond this, people with disabilities have been denied access to many of the goods of the society that the non-disabled population takes for granted. This includes shopping centers, cinemas, restaurants, university classes, employment, and leisure activities.[7]

In the 1980s, disability activists around the world began to demand equal rights for people with disabilities. A grass-roots civil rights movement led to the enactment of the *Americans With Disabilities Act* in the USA and legislation designed to achieve a fairer society for people with disabilities being passed through the Federal Parliament in Australia.[8] The Australian law, the *Disability Discrimination Act 1992*, says nothing about religion per se, but places the rights of people with disabilities clearly on the agenda of all Australian organizations and institutions.[9] It is in this setting that the community has slowly become aware of the problems facing people with disabilities, and there have been some attempts to improve the situation. This is not the place to discuss the strengths and weaknesses of the law or the social or political changes of recent times.[10] Instead, this article explores the way in which Judaism may play a positive role in the lives of those Australian Jews who are affected by disability.

JUDAISM AND SPIRITUALITY

Judaism teaches that the wisdom to resolve current issues can be found in ancient texts such as that cited in the opening paragraph (p. 56).[11] While there are many references in the written and oral law pertaining to disability, these are not well known, and being taken out of context, are at risk of misinterpretation. Further, there has been relatively little research pulling together the relevant texts and ideas on the subject of disability.[12] However, at the very center of Judaism there is an approach to the world, from which we can derive a Jewish perspective of disability. While it is hoped that this will be empowering to Jews with disabilities wherever they live, it may not be Jewish spirituality per se that is of help.

Before investigating this, however, the question of the relationship between Judaism and spirituality must be addressed. Ellen Umansky (1992), in her preface to *Piety, Persuasion and Friendship: A History of Jewish Women's Spirituality*, writes: "Jewish spirituality, like many other forms of spirituality, could be seen as an expression of individual and/or communal yearning towards the divine and a life of holiness" (p. 1).

Despite this definition, the concept of spirituality is employed throughout the book to describe the search for Jewish identity, undertaken by women over four centuries.[13] For the most part, spirituality is seen as a journey of discovery for those who have grown up in a secular culture, which they had assumed to be their own. Awakened to their Jewish roots by experiences such as anti-Semitism, the contributors to the collection describe how a renewed commitment to Judaism gave new meaning to their lives and reunited their split identities.[14]

If we are to understand Jewish spirituality as the search for, or fulfillment of, Jewish identity, a person with a disability is as likely, or unlikely, as any other to engage in the process of resolving what it means for them to be Jewish. However, the search for a Jewish identity may take a number of forms. It may be that the search relates to family history, to new social associations, to engagement in adult education, or in a commitment to the State of Israel. None of these paths is of a religious nature per se, and none could be thought of as relating to spirituality. Further, it is possible for a person to want to become more religious without engaging anything that could be thought of as spiritual. For example, one may decide to keep *Kosher* (the Jewish dietary laws) or follow the rituals associated with Jewish festivals for entirely social reasons; being 'more Jewish' is not the same as being 'more spiritual.'

Spirituality is not often thought of as being central to Jewish thought or practice. Our scriptures, which comprise the Talmud, are about rules and statutes, commandments and authority. The greater tradition, which includes both the written and oral law, consists of stories and examples of how a Jew should live her life, and Jewish responses to the lived experience of joy and sorrow, of discrimination and suffering, of pain and the harsh reality of life. For a religious Jew, the solution to most problems is not found in an ethereal spiritual world, but in people and relationships.[15] The key to spirituality in Judaism is not simply to be found in the relationship between man and Hashem (literally, the name, *Hashem* refers to the Jewish God) but, instead, is located in the relationship of man to the material world. Arthur Green defines Jewish spirituality as "life in the presence of God" or "the cultivation of a life in the ordinary world bearing the holiness once associated with sacred space and time, with temple and with holy days" (cited in Umansky, 1992, p. 1). As such, Jewish spirituality involves imbuing the material world around us with meaning, and seeking the divine in the ordinary.[16] A 'spiritual' Jew is one who sees or, rather, finds the hand of Hashem in the objects and experiences of everyday living.[17]

For religious Jews, prayer and ritual are the governing forces of life. However, there is an unhappy tendency for observant Jews to be more concerned about acting within the letter of the law than appreciating its underlying spirit; thereby reducing Jewish religiosity to external behavior. Rabbi Abraham Joshua Heschel recognized this tendency and commented that "there are Jews who are more concerned with a blood spot on an egg (which renders it *unkosher*; that is, unfit to eat under Jewish dietary laws) than with a blood spot on a dollar bill" (cited in Telushkin, 1991, pp. 417-18). What this means is that the way in which Jews behave is not necessarily a reflection on Judaism, and this is true whether the Jews in question are ultra-Orthodox, Modern Orthodox, Conservative, or Reform. The fact that Jews do not consistently live up to the ethical principles of Judaism does not detract from those principles.[18] Nor does it change the expectation of the Torah that Jews fulfil the mission of *Tikkun HaOlam*–healing the world–through the performance of *Mitzvot* (literally, commandments; colloquially, good deeds), social justice, and the positive exercise of free choice.[19]

A Jew may seek meaning in the experience of disability, but it is more likely that he or she will see no connection between being disabled and being Jewish. If anything, committed Jews with disabilities are likely to be concerned about how to deal with the barriers that limit their inclusion not only in the general Australian community but also in the Jewish community. For many, the only connection with the Jewish community comes from the possibility of help from Jewish welfare agencies or from frustrated attempts to participate in Jewish education, youth groups, swimming clubs, communal activities or synagogues. In this case, being Jewish and being disabled are simply two facts of life.

The other side of the coin relates to those who have responsibility for a disabled person. In Jewish law, this is not only the parent or the carer but also the whole community. There are rules about visiting the sick and about the treatment of people with disabilities; although these rules may not govern people in their day-to-day activities. For most Jews, even the most religious, spirituality plays an almost non-existent role in the manner in which they treat people with disabilities. Yet there are times when an event involving a person with a disability is incredibly moving, and one cannot help but feel the divine presence of Hashem.

NATAN'S STORY [20]

One of the most important events in the life of the Jew is the ceremony marking the coming of age: the time at which a young person takes on adult religious obligations. Different communities have different requirements and different ways of ensuring that rites of passage are significant. Because Judaism is a complex mixture of culture and religion, the manner of celebration of the *Bar Mitzvah* and *Bat Mitzvah* varies in place and time, from community to community. In communities in the free world, where Jews are free to exercise and enjoy their religious heritage, the Bar or Bat Mitzvah involves some sort of religious celebration as well as a formal or informal party held in the young person's honor. In Orthodox communities, a boy will be called to read from the Torah; in Reform communities, the same will be expected of a girl. The Jewish legal requirements make no distinction between children in terms of disability,[21] so the extent to which *all* children in a community are able and expected to perform the rite of passage is one means of measuring the way in which children with disabilities are included in that community. This is particularly so because in no Australian community are the requirements for a Bar or Bat Mitzvah so fixed that there is an expectation that every child will perform, learn, recite, read in the same manner as any other child. The process is sufficiently flexible to allow Synagogue communities to regularly make accommodations where they are needed in order for *any* child, independent of cultural background, social or economic status, or disability, to become bar or bat mitzvah.

Natan is a young Australian Jew who has significant psychosocial and behavioral problems associated with autism.[22] I felt honored to have been included in his Bar Mitzvah. The service was held on a Saturday at the Sephardi Synagogue in Melbourne, Victoria. When I arrived at the beginning of the service, I parted from my husband and son, and climbed the stairs to the women's section. Sitting with the mother of the bar-mitzvah boy, waves of pleasure and a great peace swept over me. While the service progressed, Natan wandered around the Synagogue. As he approached each man, he was beckoned closer; with a demonstration of care, and perhaps love, each man made a point of ensuring that Natan was at ease. Someone straightened his tie, another folded down the collar of his shirt, and yet another replaced Natan's *tallis* (prayer shawl) which had begun to trail on the ground. For maybe an hour, the men of the community not only welcomed Natan into their midst but made him feel that he had a place in that Synagogue. No-one hesitated to show his involvement in the young man's development. And everyone among the men felt that Natan's day was as important to them as it was to Natan himself.

Had I witnessed nothing more than Natan's obvious inclusion in the Synagogue community, this would have been enough for me, a Jewish human rights and disability activist, to have been proud to be an Australian Jew. When the time came for the formal part of the Bar Mitzvah, Natan made his way to the *Bimah* (the elevated platform from which the Torah is read). In a clear voice, Natan pronounced the Hebrew blessings and read his portion. This is as much as many Australian bar-mitzvah boys do, and had Natan remained and watched others continue the service, it would have been no shame. However, Natan read on, hardly stumbling or faltering as he went. At one stage it was as if the button was switched off, and Natan paused for breath. Then he started again and continued at full pelt until he reached the end. The unusual choice of a place to stop and the speed of the delivery were the only hints of Natan's disability. The rocking, which may have suggested autism to some, could also have been an exaggerated version of the rocking of religious Jews at prayer.

The celebrations began after the service and continued the next day, when many guests were invited to Natan's home to join the family at the Bar Mitzvah party. During the afternoon, Natan wandered through the house and garden. He accosted guests with some unusual questions, moved awkwardly backwards and forwards, and exhibited some rather odd behavior. Yet when the time came for him to deliver his speech, he rose to the occasion. In the speech, which he had mostly written himself (and had typed out on the computer completely on his own), Natan included the expected acknowledgements as well as a *D'var Torah*, an analysis of the portion of the Torah he had read that morning. This points to a level of learning and understanding way beyond the reach of most Australian Jewish children. It certainly is not required, but it is what one would expect from the son of a religiously learned household. The fact that Natan's autism is extremely disabling, and the fact that he has been unable to learn in the normal environment of school, did not deter him from achieving at the highest level. The fact that he had been included in the Synagogue, where he was a regular, made an enormous difference.

Of course, the credit for Natan's achievement is not his alone. From the time when recognition of his difference became unavoidable, Natan's parents sought to ensure that he would have the skills he needed to be an Orthodox Jew; the same skills as those that his brother was expected to acquire. The first question his father asked the doctors was not "can he be cured?" or "will he ever be able to do anything?" but, "will he be able to do his Bar Mitzvah?" The first words Natan spoke clearly and correctly were the words of a prayer that his older brother was hesitating to recite. For a child with autism, religious Jewish practice is in many ways easy, because with ritual and prayer comes repetition. However, because Natan's parents believed in him, they put effort not just into achieving ordinary skills like walking and talking, which the rest of us take for granted, but also into learning. An extract of Natan's father's speech gives a flavor of this:

> Many, many times you ask me the same question, "When will I be able to stop learning?"
>
> My reply is "Never." To achieve, to do something in life, you must keep learning forever.
>
> If you want to be a plumber (or a sprinkler man) you have to learn maths.
>
> You showed us yesterday at the Synagogue what a fantastic job you did in learning your Maftir and Haftorah.[23] You put the effort (with the Rabbi's help) to learn the notes so you could sing.
>
> You learnt to read Hebrew very well and fluently.
>
> You put it all together with practice.
>
> Your parents, family, and everybody at the Synagogue were proud of you. Our friends, everyone at the Synagogue, admired your effort.
>
> If you keep learning both Jewish and secular subjects, you will be able to do anything you want.
>
> Just reach for it and you will succeed.
>
> Natan, we all love you.

Natan's autism will remain a fact of his life, and the struggle to overcome all the issues that confront a young person in this position will continue throughout his life. It is hard to know whether Natan's experience of his Bar Mitzvah was spiritual in nature–it may or may not have been. But for those who have watched Natan from infancy, both the mere fact of his inclusion in the Synagogue and the incredible competence and achievement he demonstrated seemed nothing short of miraculous. Natan is not a savant–an autistic person who is a genius in some particular area–but an ordinary (or extra-ordinary) young man who worked incredibly hard over an extended period to fulfill his parents' dream.

If we were led to believe that the weekend of the Bar Mitzvah was a reflection of Natan's everyday experiences, we would be very disappointed. During the Bar Mitzvah Natan was the center of attention, just as every other child is at his or her coming of age ceremony, so his different behaviors and quirks of character were indulged and even celebrated. It would be easy, then, to suggest that Judaism accommodates people with disabilities and finds a way of being inclusive.[24] However, this has not been the experience of Jews with disabilities. The test of true inclusion in the community cannot be based on special occasions; rather, it must be measured by the lived day-to-day experiences of ordinary people who happen to have disabilities.

Judaism has not provided Natan with the level of acceptance that any of us would be happy to experience. Natan's parents wanted a complete Jewish education for their son, but their attempts to have Natan included in the Jewish school attended by his brother was unsuccessful.[25] Given that Natan's family is able to provide their children with a religious Jewish home life, Natan is more needy of friends than of religion. A number of young people were invited to Natan's Bar Mitzvah celebrations; yet this was not reciprocated. Natan is very aware and disappointed that he does not get asked to social events by his peers, such as parties or informal get-togethers, like his brother does. Inclusion in the formal synagogue community has not flowed on to inclusion in the broader community in which he lives. Natan does not understand why this is so, and is, not surprisingly, hurt and confused.

While many of us may share Natan's pain of exclusion, on one level, understanding the exclusion is easy. Natan is different: *He does not fit in*; *He does not relate to people in the same way as others*; *He is odd*; *He is an embarrassment*; *It is too hard*; *We can't manage*; *No offence meant* (of course).

On another level, understanding exclusion is difficult. Natan lives in, and his family is part of, a religious Jewish community. Members of this community take Judaism seriously. They do not work on *Shabbat* (the Jewish Sabbath): among other things, they do not drive, cook, earn money, play music or carry anything or push prams outside a carefully defined area.[26] They keep *Kosher*, they go to Synagogue regularly, and pray at home or on the road. They follow all the rituals associated with Jewish life; yet they ignore the clear ethical principles governing relationships with all people, including those with disabilities.

DISABILITY, RELIGION, AND JUDAISM

At a fundamental level, disability poses a threat to one's sense of self and, often, also to one's identity. Having a child with a disability, acquiring disability through accident or illness, being born with a genetic disorder that may be or become disabling, or becoming disabled as a result of war or age–whatever the source of the disability–it will be necessary to come to terms with limitations inherent to the disability and to an understanding of those limitations which are socially constructed. In many cases it is the social barriers to inclusion that are harder to manage than the medical or other limitations arising in the context of the body. This may be the case whether the social limitations take the form, for example, of steps making physical access impossible or the form of unfounded assumptions about competence.

It is the common experience of humankind that when confronted by such a situation, answers and comfort are sought in religion. One turns to religion to seek reassurance that everything is or will be okay, or, at least, that the treatment received from others is wrong. If a person is Jewish, he or she is also likely to look to Jewish wisdom as one possible route towards resolution of the problem.

There are two matters that are of fundamental importance to people with disabilities. The first of these is the issue of their entitlement to equality and rights. An individual may need reassurance that they are as good as everyone else and that she or he is as worthy and as valuable as any other member of the community. The second matter is the practical manifestation of equality: inclusion. People with disabilities need not just reassurance that they are entitled to the benefits of living in Australia, they also need to experience full participation in all aspects of society. For this to happen, the community as a whole must take responsibility for removing barriers and welcoming (or even celebrating) differences between people. Further, the community must demonstrate this by making whatever adjustments may be required to facilitate inclusion.

The questions we must now turn to are: Does Judaism offer reassurance that people with disabilities are valued and are entitled to be treated with dignity and respect? and, Does Judaism promote and/or require the inclusion of people with disabilities in the community? In my attempt to respond to these questions, I have drawn on the *Halacha*, the Jewish law, which literally means "the way on which one goes." There is no doubt in my mind that Judaism contains principles and rules for daily living that answer both the questions in the affirmative, and that these principles and rules have the potential to empower people with disabilities.

VALUING PEOPLE WITH DISABILITIES

While it is true that deformed babies are no longer exposed as a matter of course, people with disabilities receive the message time and again that they are worthless and a strain on or a waste of resources. My own experience of being told that I should *give up my child, forget she was ever born, get on with my life and have other children* is not unique. Other parents have reported instances such as the refusal to perform urgently needed surgery on a baby because *the shorter the life of a disabled child the better,* and the refusal to administer anesthetic because *children with Down's Syndrome do not feel pain.* These responses demonstrate the almost total devaluation of the lives of people with disabilities.

Lives Not Worth Living

The view that disabled lives are not worth living has a number of current manifestations. Dominant among these is the position that killing people with disabilities may be both morally and legally permissible. Acceptance of mercy killing and euthanasia are wide-spread, justified by the view that no rational person could possibly want to live his or her life if marred by the existence of a disability, and that, given the option, she or he would rather be dead. While a person may think that they would rather be dead than live in a particular state, this is rarely the position they adopt on reaching that state.[27] The question of whether the person consented to die, and the murderers were simply assisting suicide, is certainly not provable once the person is dead. However, where euthanasia is legal, as it is in the Northern Territory in Australia, a cloud hangs over all people with disabilities. Whenever a decision is made that the life in question is not worth living (and, given the attitude of many to people with disabilities, this could often be assumed to be the case), the person could and possibly should be 'assisted' to end his or her life.[28]

This issue is not hypothetical, but one of the so-called moral dilemmas faced by those involved in the care of sick and elderly people. Medical practitioners are called upon to authorize or carry out the 'treatment'; lawyers and judges to legitimize or de-legitimize the action. The *Latimer* case,[29] involving the murder of 12-year-old Tracy by her father, illustrates the issue. Tracy had cerebral palsy, and her father made the decision that his was a *mercy killing* because his daughter's *life was not worth living.* When charged with murder in 1994, Latimer became a celebrity and gained widespread support for his action, from the community in which he lived. Throughout the trial and his conviction in 1996 for second-degree murder, there has been a massive amount of support for Latimer, with a number of groups lobbying for his release and exoneration. People feel that the 'burden' of a child with a disability is too great for anyone to bear, and that in the circumstances, murder was justified.[30] The judges in the Canadian Supreme Court had no trouble recognizing murder and sentencing Latimer accordingly.

Lives Worth Living

The response of Judaism to mercy killings, euthanasia, assisted-suicide, and assumptions that there could be *any* life that is not worth living, is clear. All life is of the *utmost value*, and this is so whether or not disability is involved. Judaism recognizes that all people are of equal, infinite and ultimate value; even though people vary considerably in ability, personality, shape, and size. Life is a gift, to be treated with respect. Nothing could be more valuable, and no-one is less valuable.[31]

Further, Judaism removes the so-called moral dilemmas over from the realm of human decision-making, thereby relieving the doctor, lawyer, relative, etc., of the burden of making life-and-death decisions. As Kolatch (1985) comments: "Jewish tradition places the decision of who shall live and who shall die in God's hands alone. A Jew does not own her body so has no right to play with life and death" (p. 176).

Jewish law includes many principles to support the equal, infinite and ultimate value of every person. The most significant of these are the *Requirement to Choose Life* and the *Life Saving Principle*.

The Requirement to Choose Life

Jewish law requires that not only should we, at all costs, preserve life, but also that we must make an active commitment to choose life. This is derived from the Biblical Ordinance: "I have set before you life and death, blessing and curse. Choose life so that you and your offspring may live" (Deuteronomy 30:19). The interpretation of this rule is that there is no higher priority than actively choosing life–one's own as well as that of others. Abraham (1996) writes that the obligation to choose life contains the requirement that we are to value life just as Hashem does.

> The value of life is infinite and therefore the value of every part of it, however brief, is similarly infinite. . . . Once one denies the value of human life because of the nearness of death, one destroys the absolute value of all life and gives it instead a relative value only–in relation to age, health, further use to the community or any other factor one wishes to consider. *The moment one is willing to shorten life by however little, the life of a dying patient, on the grounds that it is of no further value, one destroys the infinite value of all human life.* . . . Thus, even if death is near and absolutely certain, the life of a patient is still of infinite and inestimable value, and shortening it is no way different from killing an absolutely healthy individual. (pp. 193-4) (emphasis added)

The Life Saving Principle

The Life Saving Principle is perhaps the most important of all Jewish laws, as it requires that all other Jewish laws be suspended when human life is at stake.[32] The principle is that one must do whatever one possibly can to preserve life. The words of Leviticus 18: 5, "you shall, therefore, keep my statutes and my ordinances, which if a man do he shall live by them," have been interpreted by the Rabbis to mean "you shall live by them, not die by them" (Talmud Bavli, Yoma 85b). As such, life is the most valuable attribute of all. Life comes before all other principles, and we must do all within our powers to preserve life.

Rabbi Abraham J. Heschel considers the Life Saving Principle as the mark of humanity, since the obligation to save life is uniquely human:

> The human being is being *sui generis*. The only adequate way to grasp its meaning is to think of man in human terms. Human is more than a concept of fact; it is a category of value, of the highest of all values available to us.

> What is the worth of an individual man? According to a rabbinic dictum, 'he who saves one man is regarded as if he saved all men; he who destroys one man is regarded as if he destroyed all men.' In terms of statistics, one individual is an exceedingly insignificant specimen compared with the totality of the human species. So why should the life and dignity of an individual man be regarded as infinitely precious? . . . [because every] human being is a disclosure of the Divine. (Cited in Freeman & Abrams, 1999, p. 231)

This follows from the fact that all humans are made in the image of Hashem (Genesis 1:27). Because Hashem does not have a physical form, it is diversity of types that must constitute the human manifestation of Hashem's image.[33] There have been and are people with disabilities in every society, so their presence is not aberrant but ordinary. As such, the wide variety of human forms–ranging from 'beautiful' to 'ugly,' 'physically unblemished' to 'physically marked,' from 'whole' to 'decrepit'–should all be considered as expressions of the infinite manifestations of Hashem's image.

The Life Saving Principle further confirms that every life, no matter where in the spectrum of lives, is a life worth living. Telushkin (1991) explains that, as a consequence, saving many lives at the expense of one innocent life is not permitted; by definition, many infinities cannot be worth more than one infinity (p. 530). The principle does not allow for any distinction to be made between people, as *all* life is infinite. This clearly applies to people with disabilities as well as members of the non-disabled population.

Comparing Approaches

Jewish Law does not allow mercy killing or euthanasia, but there is one situation where a person may be justified in taking the life of another. Known as the *Law of the Pursuer*, killing in self-defense in no way undermines the Life Saving Principle. The events recounted in Sanhedrin 72a demonstrate the extent of this principle:

> In fourth century Babylon a man came to Rabbi Rava and said: "The Governor of my town has ordered me to murder someone (who is innocent), and has warned me that if I do not do so he will have me killed" (can I murder the man to save my life?). Rava refused permission: "Let yourself be killed but do not kill him. Who says your blood is redder? Perhaps the blood of that man is redder." In other words, on what basis can a person argue that he is more worthy of living than his intended and innocent victim? However, Rabbi Rava would have permitted him to kill the Governor, because the Talmud teaches "he who comes to kill you, kill him first." (Cited in Telushkin, 1991, p. 507)

An understanding of this law is crucial for a Jewish resolution of a matter which has recently received enormous media attention. In 2001, the English courts were called upon to determine the appropriateness or otherwise of separating conjoined twins, Jodie and Mary. A similar case is discussed in the Talmud (Talmud Bavli, Menachot 37a), and in 1977 Rabbi Moshe Feinstein was called upon to give a ruling in a case in Philadelphia.

Rabbi Shraga Simmons compares Rabbi Feinstein's Talmudic logic with that of the British High Court and Court of Appeal.[34] While the conclusions are the same–both authorized separation–the English courts' decision-making process was unacceptable to Jewish law. In that case, Judge Robert Johnson said that:

> So killing Mary–by stopping delivery of Jodie's blood–would be an act of euthanasia, like withdrawing food and water from a terminally ill patient. If they stayed together, the few months of Mary's life would be hurtful and mean nothing to her.

So, in English law, it was permissible to kill Mary because that would be an act of kindness, for her life was not worth living. Rabbi Feinstein could not accept that killing Mary was legitimate on the basis of the potential quality of her life. Instead, he adopted the 'choose life' principle. He took seriously the reality that without surgery both twins would die. Further, there was one twin who could be saved, and another who couldn't survive separation. Rabbi Feinstein took into account the fact that one baby had no independent ability to survive and the other baby could survive on her own, but while remaining joined to her sister. As one baby's life threatened the survival of the other twin, this baby could be killed using the law of the pursuer. The law of the pursuer permits a person to stop and kill the pursuer where the pursuer is directly threatening to kill another person, even if the threat to life is unintentional. In this case one baby posed a threat to the other's survival, and, in order to choose life, that threat must be removed.

EQUALITY OF PEOPLE WITH DISABILITIES

Disability as Punishment

Even if we accept that people with disabilities are as valuable and as entitled to life as those without disabilities, the question remains as to why some people have disabilities and others do not. Is disability somehow a fallen state? And has the media got it right when people with disabilities are portrayed as morally deviant, morally depraved and morally deformed? Should the birth of a child with some sort of disability be grounds for mourning rather than celebration? Is someone to blame for the disability? Is disability a reflection on or of the person's immorality? Is disability a punishment for wrongdoing, or a burden that some people must bear because they have sinned?

The dominant position in Jewish thinking is that disability is not a punishment for sin (Kolatch, 1985, p. 64; Telushkin, 1991, p. 504). Judaism rejects the idea of original sin, and believes that all people are born with the capacity to do both good and evil. We all have the inclination to do good (*yetzer hatov*) and the inclination to do evil (*yetzer hara*). From a Jewish perspective, it is the choices we make and our responses to these impulses, particularly resisting the *yetzer hara*, which ultimately determine who we are.[35] However, having the capacity to exercise free will makes it inevitable that every person will make both good and bad decisions. Being human, and therefore far from perfect, results in people often making wrong choices (Kushner, 2001, pp. 52-53). As such, Judaism rejects the possibility that Hashem would punish people for simply being human. The dilemma of good people suffering and bad people prospering is not important for our purposes, although the enormous Jewish literature on this point may give some comfort to those whose disability involves chronic illness or ongoing pain.[36] What is important is that from a Jewish perspective there is no moral deviance attached to being a person with a disability.[37]

Equality or Inferiority

Removing sin from the disability equation leaves open the question of status, stigma and the ascription of inferiority so often attributed to people with disabilities. From a Jewish perspective, however, no one is entitled to judge another and no one is entitled to conclude that their own "blood is redder." As Abraham (1996) comments:

> We have no yardstick by which to measure the worth and importance of a life, not even in terms of the person's knowledge of Torah and the fulfillment of Mitzvot. One must set aside the Shabbat laws even for a person who is old and sick, who may be socially unacceptable because of a repulsive external disease, who may be mentally retarded and incapable of performing any Mitzvot. (p. 195)

This analysis is consistent with the frequent references in Jewish texts to the ultimate and equal value of all people. At the very beginning of the Bible, we are told that Hashem created only one human, Adam. Rabbi Perl comments that among the reasons for this is that:

> . . . each person has the value of a world and that unlike when man mints a coin, with each coin identical to the original mold, each person has similar features to Adam, but at the same time, each human being is unique. Thus, each human being has infinite value and is also unique.[38]

Further, Rabbi Perl argues that "since this Mishna never qualifies or limits to which type of human beings it is referring, it clearly means that each and every person created has the same infinite value, just as each and every person is unique."[39] Importantly, for our purposes, he continues:

> Thus, each developmentally disabled person indeed has infinite value in Judaism and has the same value as any other person. The obligation to violate the Shabbat and save a life applies equally to developmentally disabled people as well as to anyone else. Similarly, the obligation to save the life of someone in danger applies equally to developmentally disabled people as to any other person, as the Talmud makes no distinctions. This is why developmentally disabled males over the age of bar mitzvah are counted for a minyan. Similarly, the Shulchan Aruch rules that parents of a developmentally challenged child have fulfilled their obligation for procreation like any other parents.[40]

Siegel makes a similar point: "If all humanity does have a common origin, it is obvious, then, that the disabled or handicapped are not derived from an alien source which is 'inferior,' since all have a common source."[41] He points out that when the earth is flooded, and all of those not on the Ark perished, there is again a single root of renewed humanity through the offspring of Mr and Mrs Noah. The Rabbis agree that another lesson one can learn from the singular creation of Adam is that arguments about superiority of lineage do not hold. No-one is entitled to tell another, "'my father was greater than yours,' since all human beings are descended from one father" (Telushkin, 1991, p. 529).

The Golden Rule

The day-to-day application of accepting the moral equivalence and infinite value of every individual can be found in what is known as the *Golden Rule*, "Love your neighbour as yourself, I am the Lord" (Leviticus 19:18).

Because we are all made in Hashem's image, we must treat each other with dignity and respect. The Baal Shem Tov placed emphasis on the requirement that we love ourselves, and suggested that "just as we love ourselves, despite the faults we know we have, so should we love our neighbors despite the faults we see in them." Further, just as the Jewish people were strangers in the land of Egypt, we know what it is like to be treated as an outsider (Exodus 23:9). How to treat others is a direct result of our own experience; Hillel's formulation is "do not do unto others what you would not want others to do to you" (Talmud Yerushalmi Shabbat 31a.).

Rabbi Akiva considered the Golden Rule to be the major principle of the Jewish law (Talmud Yerushalmi, Nedarim 9:4) (Telushkin, 1991, p. 63). If, instead of respecting others, we treat them badly–abuse them, discriminate against them, shame them–we not only disobey the Golden Rule but we also bring shame upon ourselves. Because we were all made in the image of Hashem, Jewish teaching holds that:

> . . . when you shame another human being, whom are you shaming? It is the image of the Holy One Blessed be He. And a person who does not think this way is considered as if the divine image is not resting upon him![42]

The Jewish Hero

The equality and worth of all people, with or without disabilities, can be demonstrated by reference to biblical history, where many of the leaders were disabled in some way. Sarah and Rachel were barren: a serious limitation for women at the time; Isaac was blind in his old age, and Leah had a visual disability; Jacob had a club foot, and was described as a "simple man," possibly suggesting an intellectual disability; Isaac was also not as we'd expect–at the age of 10 or 11, he allowed his father to bind him to the stake and would have co-operated in his own sacrifice had Hashem not intervened.

Abrams (1998) is mistaken when she takes the High Priest to be the Jewish 'ideal type.'[43] It is true that the expectation of a High Priest is that he (never she) would be pure and unblemished. This is a condition of entry to the Holy-of-Holies, where Hashem's presence could be felt and where direct communication with Hashem was possible. There are two responses that must be made. The first is that, overall, the High Priest does not play a very significant role in Jewish belief or action. This is particularly so since the destruction of the second Temple. Children who study at Jewish schools do not even learn of the High Priest until quite late in the piece. On the other hand, they will know a substantial amount about the specific characteristics of the Matriarchs and Patriarchs, from quite a young age.

The second response to placing the High Priest as a prototype of a Jewish hero is even more important. While the High Priests could not approach Hashem, except in extremely limited circumstance, the Patriarchs, judges and prophets (some of whom, such as Ehud Ben Gera whose right hand was withered, had a disability) spoke directly to and even argued with Hashem.

Perhaps the best example of a hero, and a preferable prototype of a Jewish hero, is Moses. He was the greatest leader of the People of Israel and was referred to with the highest praise as *Rabaynu*, our teacher; this was of a higher status than that given to a Patriarch, who was referred to as *Avinu*, our father. Moses had a speech impediment which greatly affected his self-confidence. He told Hashem that he could not speak with Pharaoh, and that Hashem should send his brother Aaron, whose 'silver tongue' would be a far better match. Hashem sent Moses, disability and all, to confront Pharaoh and to lead the Children of Israel out of Egypt. Hashem instructed Moses to climb Mt Sinai; despite his disability, Moses came face to face with Hashem and lived to tell the tale. The message is very clear. People with disabilities can be ordinary members of the community; but they can also be extra-ordinary members of the community. Hashem could not be convinced that a person with a disability was inferior. If this is unacceptable for Hashem, how much more so must this be for mere mortals.

In an examination of Jewish history, in particular during the period of the Torah and the Rabbis, Siegel finds:

What is particularly significant is that, in any instance in the Jewish tradition, be it in the interpretation of homilies, in the description of heroes,
in the legislative category, at no point is there denigration of the individual with a disability, or humor (cruel or otherwise) at the expense of this
individual, or exclusion of the individual from the community as a total
segregate, or a description for the handicapped individual as one who is
cursed of God (*or*, for that matter, a demi-God or select of God). Disabled or not, the individual is a human being.[44]

This confirms that people with disabilities are no different from anyone else
in the eyes of Hashem, and, as a direct consequence, should be no different
from anyone else in human terms.

THE LAW OF INCLUSIVE SOCIAL RELATIONS

As we have seen, Judaism is unequivocal in its acceptance of people with
disabilities. Jewish law demands that people with disabilities be treated as
equal members of the community. The lives of people with disabilities must be
valued, and the experience of disability taken to be irrelevant to the entitlement to be treated with equal concern, dignity and respect. What this means in
practical terms is that to be consistent with Jewish law, society must be designed and/or structured in a manner consistent with equality.

For this to occur, Judaism provides an ethical framework for ensuring that
all social relations are inclusive. A primary aspect of this is education. If we
are not taught how to respect difference, we may not be able to act respect-
fully. If we don't know that people with disabilities are ordinary members of
the community, and that having a disability does not lower one's status and
does not devalue the person, it will be easy to accept the general view presented in the media and secular society that disabled lives are not worth living
and that people with disabilities are morally deviant.

The education about people with disabilities will need to include discussion
of the many principles of Judaism relating to the way the community should
respond to disability. These principles are designed to maintain the harmony
and the dignity of human beings, one to another. A crucial element of this is
recognizing the person first and the disability as one of very many characteristics. Reducing a person to the disability, or thinking of the person as a medical
category, is disrespectful of the person. Further, focusing on a person's limitations rather than on their personality or ability will generally have the effect of
devaluing the person. Adopting a flexible rather than rigid approach to religious practice will result in a fairer society, where inclusion is a matter of
course and exclusion is carefully thought through before it happens.

One aspect of Natan's story (p. 60) is the relative ease with which Natan was accepted into the formal aspects of Jewish religious practice. Had he been unable to read or sing, ways would have been found to allow him to perform his Bar Mitzvah. The same is true where girls are concerned. I had the honor of participating in the Bat Mitzvah of Tova.[45] Tova has severe multiple disabilities which result in her being unable to speak, read or write. She requires one-on-one care and very easily becomes distressed in crowds. Her Bat Mitzvah was a very important achievement and another extremely moving occasion. Tova knew it was her special day, and that everybody there had come especially for her. With the ceremony being conducted in a Reform synagogue, the female Rabbi played the guitar and sang much of the service, which was specifically designed for Tova. A *Tallis* was placed on Tova's shoulders, and a prayer was said by her parents. Her brothers, aunts, and uncles participated in the service, which was kept extremely brief to meet Tova's needs. Although much that happened that morning was quite foreign to an Orthodox Jew, I felt privileged to have been invited to the Bat Mitzvah. And, once again, I was proud that a way was found for Tova to celebrate and be celebrated. Both Natan's and Tova's parents worked extremely hard to make the events happen and be meaningful. Hopefully, other parents will follow these examples.

While inclusion in the formal aspects of Judaism is very important, it represents only a small part of Jewish life. The importance of bringing inclusion to other aspects of the Jewish life of people with disabilities cannot be understated. The principles of Jewish law that are pertinent to an inclusive society include the *Stumbling Block Principle*, the rules related to *Visiting the Sick*, the laws of *Justice* and *Charity*, and the *Principle of Inclusive Education*. When these principles are read together, it will become clear that the problems that confront people with disabilities go well beyond bodily limitations. Rather, socially constructed barriers to inclusion cause much of the frustration felt by people with disabilities. This means that the broader community will need to be proactive in removing barriers, as well as ethical in all its interactions with people with disabilities.

> In Leviticus 19, for the first time in history, we are called upon to create a new chapter in our relations with those who are disabled. We are told that they deserve honor, respect, and the facilities they require. We are informed that they merit attention and care and that they will receive God's love and protection. That is why the verse ends with the words "You shall fear your God." Just because a person may think that the deaf will not hear a curse or the blind will not see an insulting gesture, we must remember that God hears and sees on their behalf and in the end, the tormentors will receive their just punishment.[46] (Weider)

The Stumbling Block Principle

The Stumbling Block Principle is often considered to be the most basic expression of Jewish values. This principle comes from the biblical text:

> You shall not curse the deaf nor put a stumbling block before the blind, but you shall fear the Lord your God. (Leviticus 19:14)

Cursed Be He Who Misleads the Blind (Deuteronomy 27:18)

On one level, this law can be taken literally, and analogies can be drawn. Judaism forbids insulting those who cannot hear and blocking the path of the blind. In each case, one is actively creating barriers which limit the participation of people with disabilities in the society. This recognizes that what restricts a person with a disability from functioning as a full member of the society is not only the disability itself. It is also the natural and artificial barriers, which we see all around us, which interfere with the ability to function fully in society. This ancient ruling is an articulation of the social model of disability, which focuses attention away from the individual pathology. Instead of assuming that a medical description of the individual's disability accounts for his or her failure to be actively included in society (the medical model of disability), the biblical law asks the non-disabled population to ensure that they are not responsible for creating stumbling blocks. On this point, Daniel Taub notes that:

> . . . the commandment also has broader social applications. Thus, planning city developments without taking into consideration the needs of the disabled (ramps for wheelchairs, traffic lights with beepers for the blind) could literally be creating a 'stumbling block.' (Cited in Telushkin, 2000, p. 87)

This recognizes the role of the community in engaging in exclusionary practices and in *creating* social and physical barriers to the full inclusion of people with disabilities. Modern examples of this are: providing crucial information printed in ten-point type; providing transportation for the public, but not allowing guide dogs on board; showing films without captioning, to exclude a deaf person from joining his or her family at the movies; or housing government offices in a building with no ramps or lifts.

The Stumbling Block Principle also encapsulates the Jewish perspective on what it means to be a person with a disability. Siegel argues that being forbidden to curse the deaf, who could not hear the curse anyway, involves the recognition that "one who suffers the impairment of a physical sense nevertheless is not unable to perceive." And it is important to acknowledge that "a physical impairment is not to be equated with a lack of intelligence or of understanding."[47] Equally, generalized assumptions and stereotyping of people with disabilities pose a great threat to their inclusion in the community. This tells us that the only appropriate response to disability is to take each individual as you find them.

The Jewish perspective on disability is made clear by the Stumbling Block Principle. People with disabilities are entitled to be treated with dignity and respect, and this involves seeing the whole person. They must not be subjected to exploitation or be demeaned in any way. It is the responsibility of every member of the community to refrain from erecting barriers to equality and to remove stumbling blocks as they become aware of them.[48] As these blocks may be attitudinal, Jews are also instructed to examine their own emotions and behavior, and not to sit in judgment of others.

Disability Is Not the Measles

As a general rule, people with disabilities are not ill, and have no desire to be treated as such. So wishing someone a speedy recovery is inappropriate, and is symbolic of the failure of the well-wisher to accept the person's difference. However, there are times when people with disabilities are unwell, and in these circumstances the laws pertaining to visiting the sick should be followed. Where a person's disability is chronic illness, the limitations on their ability to engage in everyday life are extremely disabling. In this situation, perhaps more importantly than in any other case, the person's ability to cope will be greatly enhanced by the rules of visiting the sick.[49]

Jewish law obliges all Jews to visit the sick. The following sliding scale concerning visiting the sick has been derived: sending a card; making a phone call; making a personal visit; visiting and taking an interest in their condition; and, most importantly, providing assistance in whatever way is helpful to the ill person. Jewish thought stresses the therapeutic effects of human interaction; such as visiting, empathic support, reinforcement of love in relationships, and a return to communal life. David Freeman and Judith Abrams (1999) have commented:

> Illness isolates; from the isolation comes depression; and from depression, comes a worsening of disease. The sages knew that visiting is more than a social courtesy; it is therapeutic. (p. xxii)

The Rabbis recognized how easily a sick person can feel abandoned and become depressed. They declared that anyone who visits a sick person removes one sixtieth of his illness (Talmud Bavli, Bava Mezia 30b), while those who stay away hasten death (Telushkin, 1991, p. 531).

Justice

Just as Judaism emphasizes action over faith, Jewish law is less concerned with feelings or emotion than it is with behavior. The rule governing all social interactions is "Justice, justice you shall pursue" (Deuteronomy 16:20).

Judaism demands the just treatment of all members of society, irrespective of how one may feel about them. This means that fear or repulsion, condescension or pity, which are common responses to different appearances or different behavior, are not an excuse for treating people with disabilities badly. Emotional responses do not excuse segregation or institutionalization, as these are clearly unjust responses to people with disabilities. Instead, justice requires that people with disabilities are included in all aspects of society. Justice means that exclusion from the informal goings on of the community, such as that experienced by Natan, is as unacceptable as any formal exclusion. Equally, ensuring informal inclusion does not justify the failure to ensure formal inclusion.

Charity

The notion of charity that is adopted by Jewish law is quite distinct from the Christian usage. The word *tzedakah*, often translated as charity, actually means justice. As such, one who gives tzedakah acts justly; one who does not acts unjustly (and contrary to Jewish law). Maimonides considers there to be eight levels of tzedakah, from giving charity grudgingly (level 8) through to anonymous donors and recipients (level 2).[50] The best form of tzedakah (level 1) is where a donor provides whatever it takes to ensure that the recipient no longer need rely on charity. Examples of tzedakah are offering a person a long-term loan to establish their own business, offering a partnership in a business, or employing the person and ensuring that the salary is sufficient to keep them out of debt. Many more competent and able people with disabilities are out of work than their non-disabled counterparts. And the cost of living is much greater for a people with disabilities, who may require expensive equipment or medication, than it is for the non-disabled. Providing free equipment for those who need it would be another exercise in tzedakah. In other words, tzedakah, in its ideal manifestation, is about empowering people by giving them the possibility of independence and self-sufficiency. Having to rely on or ask for charity is demeaning; ensuring that this is the exception and not the rule is a fundamental value of Judaism.

Education

From a Jewish point of view, the most important activity in which a person can engage is the study of Torah. Natan's father told him that being autistic is no excuse–he can never stop learning. A strong parent movement has resulted in the Jewish day-school system being one of the first in Australia to include children with disabilities, and a comparatively high percentage of Jewish children with disabilities now have access to Jewish education in Australia. But the achievement of equal treatment within the school system has a long way to go. Natan's problems were considered too great for the school he had attended to allow him to remain. Some children are allowed to attend the schools, but with no provision for their educational needs to be met. In other cases, parents have had children accepted into the school on the basis that they pay full fees and also pay for an aide. There are even cases in which the parents of a child with disabilities paid for renovations to the school to facilitate their child's attendance. There are children who have been tormented and/or excluded from mainstream activities because of their disabilities.

On the other hand, there are enough success stories for parents to still push for inclusion, and some individual children have achieved more highly than anyone would have expected. The daughter I was meant to have discarded, who is now 11, has a group of loyal friends who are all high achievers. Just as my older children have done, her friends will adapt games to suit her abilities. Socially, she has no problems, and she is competent in many ways that would seem impossible in the light of a mild-to-moderate intellectual disability. As her friends say, Eli can learn almost anything, but the way she learns is quite different from the norm. And having told some of her story, I can gloat that Eli must be the only child with an intellectual disability who has been invited to go along with her friend to a gifted and talented program.

Jewish law on the question of inclusion in mainstream education is far more advanced than one might imagine. There is story after story providing evidence that Torah was taught to individuals with intellectual and other disabilities.

> The sons of the sister of Rabbi Yochanan were clearly developmentally disabled, but, nevertheless, sat in the advanced Torah classes of Rabbi Judah, nodding their heads and moving their lips. One day Rabbi Judah prayed for their recovery, and they were miraculously cured. Then it was

found that they were totally versed in Halachah, Midrash, and the entire Talmud.[51] (Talmud Bavli, Chagiga 3a)

What this story shows us is that, first, children with disabilities should be included into age-appropriate classes, and, secondly, that people should not be so quick to judge the effect of a disability. In the case of Rabbi Judah's students, the assumption was made that unusual behaviors were evidence of lack of understanding, when in fact they were exactly the opposite. Everyone had assumed that nothing was being comprehended, based on the outward reactions of nodding. In reality they assimilated all of Rabbi Judah's teachings, but they were incapable of expressing what they had internalized. As such, developmental delay or communication disorders are no excuse to exclude a child with disabilities from the classroom. Rabbi Perl comments:

> Unless Jews are sensitive to the learning needs of all children, even the smallest minority, there is a dimension lacking in the Jewish community. Therefore, we can infer . . . that it is the obligation of the Jewish community to be sympathetic and sensitized to the Jewish and Torah needs of every segment and category of child within the Jewish community, including the developmentally disabled child . . .[52]

Being educated as a Jew will give a person the chance to become a valued member of the Jewish community. There is no reason why a person with a disability cannot count as one of the ten men needed for certain prayers,[53] and many ritual elements of Judaism do not require a high level of education. Being included in educational settings will give a child the potential to make friends and to be accepted for who she or he is. And, knowing that education does not stop at twelve or thirteen with the Bar or Bat Mitzvah, or at eighteen with finishing school, should provide the opportunity for Jews with disabilities to find many safe learning environments in which to commence or continue Jewish learning.

SPIRITUALITY AND AUSTRALIAN JEWRY

There are approximately 110,000-120,000 Jews living in Australia today. The Australian Jewish community is not just one community; rather, it is comprised of many communities, the majority of which are located in capital cities, particularly Sydney and Melbourne. There are also a number of communities and families living in smaller cities, rural and even remote areas. Religiously, Australian Jewry consists of ultra-Orthodox, modern Orthodox, Conservative and Reform Jews. Because Judaism is cultural as well as religious,[54] there are secular and non-religious Jews who nonetheless maintain a strong Jewish identity. While Jews constitute a small percentage of the Australian population, by world standards, the Jewish community is very strong. A high percentage of Jewish children attend Jewish day schools, and many others receive Jewish education at state schools or at home or both.

The profile of Australian Jewry matches and reflects that of the broader Australian community in which it is based. This means that we can expect that there will be the same prevalence of disability (18%) among Jews as non-Jews, the same incidence of domestic violence, the same problems of poverty. There are some Jewish-genetic disorders, and no doubt the exploration of the Human Genome will find many other differences relating to Jewish biological inheritance. There are Jews with physical disabilities, mental illness, visual and hearing impairment, intellectual disability and chronic illness. While medical science may improve the position of some people (and potentially ensure that people with some potential disabilities are simply not born into this world),[55] Australia's aging population will ensure that the number of people with disabilities, and hence the number of Jews with disabilities, will increase in the coming years.

It should now be clear that Judaism is potentially very empowering for people with disabilities. In Judaism, all people are entitled to being treated with dignity and respect. People with disabilities are ordinary members of the community who have as much potential as anyone else to become leaders or heroes. Biblical Jewish leaders provide role models for people with disabilities, as they, too, are portrayed as ordinary imperfect human beings, many of whom are disabled. No Jew is permitted to judge another as inferior–all life is valuable, and no-one's life is more valuable than anyone else's. If the quality of someone's life is poor, then the community must work to improve the situation. The community should take responsibility to ensure the inclusion of people with disabilities so as to allow for personal issues arising in the context of a disability to be dealt with. This is the inclusive society Judaism aspires to.

Jewish law is based on an understanding that all people have the power to exercise free will to do good or evil. Even where a person is well intentioned, the *Halacha* assumes that she or he will not automatically know how to act ethically, so rules and commandments are laid down. However, we should not assume that because a person follows the rules and rituals of Judaism relating to religious practice, that person is more important in the eyes of Hashem. One could have one's entire life dedicated to Hashem, and outwardly be as religious as could be, but nonetheless fail in the ethical treatment of people with disabilities. If this were the case, this person would be significantly hampered in his pursuit of Judaism. This is because, fundamentally, Judaism is an ethical code designed to provide guidance with respect to social interaction.

The Jewish code of ethics takes humanity or humanness to be the basic building block of society. Because all people are derived from the union of Adam and Eve, all people are not only of equal value but also of ultimate value. Perhaps the best way to understand this is to consider the Talmudic maxim that:

> . . . whoever destroys one life is considered by the Torah as if he destroyed an entire world, and whoever save one life is considered by the Torah as if he saved an entire world. (Talmud Bavli–Sanhedrin 37a)

Not only does Judaism hold that every person is of equal worth, it also considers that every moment of every life is of infinite value. This is not contingent on good health or an able body. Therefore, Judaism totally rejects the notion that some lives are not worth living.

Given this proposition, no distinction can legitimately be drawn between different lives. Men are not valued more than women; old men, more than young men; children or babies, more than adults. A person with a disability, a person who is ill, a person who could be seen as different in any way, is no less a person. This is essential to understanding Judaism's attitude to disability. While there are rules and regulations found in the Talmud that relate to any imaginable situation, and rules and regulations that both directly and indirectly concern people with disabilities, all interpretation of these rules must be read down in terms of the underlying principle of the ultimate value of all lives.

The treatment of people with disabilities within Judaism is not the same as the way in which Jews treat people with disabilities. The fact that Jews are unable to live up to the ethical principles of Judaism does not detract from those principles. The way in which Jews behave is not necessarily a reflection on Judaism, and this is true whether the Jews in question are ultra-Orthodox, modern Orthodox, Conservative or Reform. Jews who are assimilated into the broader community, and whose behavior is predominantly secular, may act more consistently with Judaism than those who appear to be religious. This may explain why people with disabilities have been excluded from Jewish communities or from the activities of the community. Jews are no more exempt from bad behavior than non-Jews. Jews, like other people, may be scared of or even horrified by those who look or behave differently.

Because people with disabilities have become more vocal members of the community, and have begun to demand to be treated with dignity and respect, the Australian Jewish community has slowly begun to be responsive to the varying needs of people with disabilities. Some positive examples of this are the installation of lifts to allow women with disabilities access to the women's galleries of Synagogues, and those with mobility impairments, access to communal buildings, and the installation of a hearing loop in Sydney's Great Synagogue. These are partly a response to the Commonwealth *Disability Discrimination Act 1992*, which proscribes discrimination on the grounds of disability. However, it could be argued that access to buildings is a prerequisite to participation for those with physical limitations. Strong parents' movements have been responsible for the increasing number of children who are included in schools and in Jewish youth groups. The presence of people with disabilities amongst Jews not only facilitates the potential spirituality of the disabled individuals but also brings about an awareness of disability, which may lead to improvements in the non-disabled population.

This does not really tackle the question of spirituality and Judaism. It may be that *mitzvot*, or good deeds, may be performed with respect to people with disabilities, but this may or may not be thought of in spiritual terms. On the other hand, if we accept that the "words we use, the charity we give, the ways we invite people into our homes, and even how we make love are all part of Jewish life's broad path to spiritual encounter," then Jews with disabilities must be given the opportunity to lead an ethically Jewish life.

It is clear, at least from the perspective developed here, that unless people with disabilities are included in the community, there is little chance that they will be able to experience anything spiritual. Jewish spirituality can only come through Jewish learning or through participation in spiritual Jewish experiences. If "the individual's way to holiness and to God is through living in relationship with others," then inclusion in the community is an essential starting point for spirituality (Gordis, 1995, p. 187).[56]

It has always been considered that a Jew should devote at least equal energy to their Jewish learning as they do to their secular learning. For people with disabilities who have been segregated and excluded from almost all aspects of life, it may be, as it was for Natan, that Jewish learning is the route to other learning. Further, for those people with disabilities who have been unable to gain employment in the broader community, or to have any sort of livelihood, establishing their spiritual livelihood through Jewish learning may be crucial to their sense of person. There is no good reason to exclude people with disabilities from Jewish life, and there are a million and one good reasons to include them. Prominent among these is that Jewish learning demands this.

NOTES

1. See M. Jones & L. Marks, *Law and people with disabilities, International encyclopaedia of the social and behavioural sciences*; Title 3.8.133; Discipline: Law, 2001.

2. See D. Mitchell & S. Snyder, *Narrative prosthesis: Disability and the dependencies of discourse*, Ann Arbor: University of Michigan Press, 2000; and H. Deutsch &

F. Nussbaum (Eds.), *'Defects': Engendering the modern body*, Ann Arbor: University of Michigan Press, 2000.

    3. See R. G. Thomson, *Extraordinary bodies: Figuring physical disability in American culture and literature*, New York: Columbia University Press, 1997.

    4. See K. Johnson, The pied piper plays again . . . the lure of contractualism, in T. Carney & A. Yeatman (Eds.), *The new contractualism*, Sydney: Federation Press, 2002.

    5. See M. Jones & L. Marks, Valuing people through law: Whatever happened to Marion, in M. Jones & L. A. B. Marks (Eds.), *Explorations on law and disability in Australia*, Special Issue of *Law in Context*, Sydney: Federation Press, 2000, pp. 147-181; and L. Chenoweth, A long road to justice: Sexual abuse of people with disabilities, in M. Jones & L. Marks (Eds.), *Disability, divers-ability and legal change*, Dordrecht: Martinus Nijhoff, 1999.

    6. See S. Cook & R. Slee, Struggling with the fabric of disablement: Picking up the threads of the law and education, in M. Jones & L. Marks (Eds.), *Disability, divers-ability and legal change*, Dordrecht: Martinus Nijhoff, 1999; and M. Jones & L. Marks, Fostering inclusive societal values through law, *International Journal of Children's Rights* (forthcoming).

    7. One example of this involved a visually impaired man who wanted equal access to tickets for the Sydney Olympic Games: *Maguire v Sydney Organising Committee for the Olympic Games* [2000] EOC 93-041; [2001] EOC pp. 93-124.

    8. While the *Americans With Disabilities Act* has been used as a model by most countries around the world, the Australian law is unique: see M. Jones & L. Marks, A bright new era of equality, independence, and freedom–Casting an Australian gaze on the ADA, in L. Francis & A. Silvers (Eds.), *Americans with disabilities*, Routledge, 2000, pp. 371-86.

    9. See L. Basser & M. Jones, The *Disability Discrimination Act*: A three dimensional approach to operationalizing human rights, *Melbourne University Law Review* (forthcoming).

    10. On the role of law in supporting the position of people with disabilities, see: M. Jones & L. Marks (Eds.), Law and the social construction of disability, *Disability, divers-ability and legal change,* Dordrecht: Martinus Nijhoff, 1999, pp. 3-24.

    11. Any discussion of a Judaic or Jewish perspective on any topic is inherently fraught. Those familiar with Judaism will be aware that there is a very wide range of ways in which Jews express and experience their Judaism. There is a religious continuum in Australia from Reform to Conservative to Modern Orthodox to Ultra Orthodox, and there are Jews whose identity is beyond religion, which is expressed by a variety of secular and cultural means. The analysis here is from a modern traditional Orthodox–mainstream–view of Judaism, which should find resonance with most practicing Jews.

    12. A beginning has been made in this regard by Judith Z. Abrams in J. Abrams, *Judaism and disability: Portrayals in ancient texts from the Tanach through the Bavli*, Washington DC: Gallaudet University Press, 1998. Abrams approaches the subject from the perspective of Reform Judaism, which has led her to quite different conclusions than I do from the perspective of Orthodoxy.

    13. Historically, women had been denied a level of Jewish education consistent with their secular education, and have been excluded from many formal aspects of Jewish practice. See A. Cantor, *Jewish women Jewish men*, San Francisco: Harper, 1995; B. Greenberg, *On women and Judaism*, Philadelphia: Jewish Publication Society of

America, 1981; and M. Meiselman, *Jewish women in Jewish Law*, New York: Ktav Publishing House, 1978.

14. Where the women are comfortable with their own identities, their comments are included to demonstrate the possibility of a holistic approach to being a woman and being Jewish.

15. See A. Kaplan, The infinite light, *The Aryeh Kaplan Anthology 1*, NCSY, 1998, pp. 110-111.

16. Rabbi Joseph Soloveitchik, the leading Orthodox scholar of our times, considers that the main tasks of *halakhic man* involve compliance with the ethical aspects of the law. In *The Man of Faith in the Modern World*, he wrote that "the Halakah operates in the practical realm of reality, and an insular withdrawal from the creative act in the pragmatic world is contrary to the spirit of the Torah." See J. Soloveitchik, *Man of faith in the modern world, vol. 2*, New Jersey: Ktav Publishing, 1989, p. 42.

17. J. H. Hertz comments: "Holiness is thus not so much an abstract or mystic idea, as a regulative principle in the everyday lives of men and women . . . Holiness is thus attained not by flight from the real world, nor by monk-like renunciation of human relationships of family or station, but by the spirit in which we fulfil the obligations of life in its simplest and commonest details: in this way–by doing justly, loving mercy, and walking humbly with God–is everyday life transfigured." (1977, p. 497). J. Telushkin, *Jewish literacy*, New York: William Morrow & Co, 1991, p. 549.

18. Rabbi Heschel commented that "among religious Jews today, disproportionate emphasis often is placed on rituals, as if Judaism's ethical laws were offered merely as advice and are not as binding as the rituals" (cited by Telushkin, 1991, p. 549).

19. The obligation of Jews "to perfect the world under the rule of God" is so important that it is reiterated in the *Aleinu* prayer, which is recited 3 times a day (Telushkin, 1991, p. 549).

20. Natan is not the true name of the young man involved, as I have changed his identity to protect the privacy of those involved. Natan means gift, and despite all that has happened in his life, Natan is a gift to those who are privileged to know him. The family is happy to be contacted, via my email address, to share their experience with others.

21. From an orthodox perspective, there is a question of whether a blind person is obliged, or even permitted, to read from the Torah (literally, the Teaching or the Constitution of Judaism, the term *Torah* generally refers to the 5 Books of the Old Testament, but is also used to refer to both the written and oral law). It is not possible, given the limitations of this paper, to deal here with issues, such as prohibitions, relating to specific disabilities. This will be the subject of another article.

22. For information about autism, see the Autism Society of America, at: http://www.autism-society.org/whatisautism/autism.html#whatisautism; Center for the Study of Autism, at: http://www.autism.org/contents.html

23. The *Maftir* is the final part of the Torah reading, which is a repetition of the last verses of that day's Reading of the Torah. However, the term actually refers to the person called up to read the concluding section of the Torah Reading. Generally the same person will read the *Haftorah*, a reading from the Book of Prophets, which usually has some connection with what has just been read from the Torah. The custom of reading the Haftorah was instituted when the ruling power forbade, usually on pain of death, the reading of the Torah itself.

24. I argue below that Judaism *does* provide for the inclusion of all members of the Jewish community, but that Jews do not often live up to the expectations of Jewish law.

25. This is not to suggest that this has been the case for all young Australian Jews. My daughter (who has an intellectual disability) has been fully and very successfully included at the Jewish school which my other 4 children have attended. This has also been the case for many other children. However, inclusion at school has not necessarily been successful socially, and many children have found themselves isolated and friendless.

26. Carrying outside the home is forbidden unless there is an *Eruv* erected. An Eruv is an artificial boundary to an area, built with string and wire, which allows Orthodox Jews to carry on Shabbat. The term *eruv* means to mix or join together, referring to the construction of the wall. The only place in Australia where there is an Eruv is in Sydney's Eastern Suburbs. On the Eruv and the law concerning people with disabilities, see F. Rosner, *Biomedical ethics and Jewish law*, New Jersey: Ktav, 2001, pp. 504-506.

27. See J. Fitzgerald, Bioethics, disability and death: Uncovering cultural bias in the euthanasia debate, in M. Jones & L. Marks (eds), *Disability, divers-ability and legal change*, Dordrecht: Martinus Nijhoff, 1999.

28. Similar issues arise in the context of prenatal testing and decisions to abort foetuses (and the Human Genome Project will provide more and more genetic markers of 'abnormality'), decisions to sterilize young women with disabilities to prevent unwanted pregnancies (rather than to prevent sexual abuse). See M. Jones & L. Marks, Valuing people through law: Whatever happened to Marion, in M. Jones & L. Marks (eds), *Explorations on law and disability in Australia*, Special Issue of *Law in Context*, Sydney, Federation Press, 2000, pp. 147-181; and M. Jones & L. Marks, The dynamic developmental model of emerging rights in children, *International Journal of Children's Rights, Vol. 2*, pp. 265-291.

29. Latimer's case can be found at *R. v. Latimer*, [2001] 1 S.C.R. 3, 2001 SCC 1.

30. There have been a number of other similar cases over the last 10 years. In the US, two mothers killed their children. The mother of the non-disabled children was labeled as a monster, and sentenced to life imprisonment; the mother of the disabled children was viewed as a saint who had done more than could be expected of her–and she was set free.

31. On this question, see Rosner (2001), pp. 223-287; Rabbi Avi Shafran (2001), *Legalizing assisted suicide* (at: http://aish.com/societywork/sciencenature/Legalizing_Assisted_ Suicide.asp); S. Bernstein, *Doctor-assisted suicide* (2001) (at: http://aish.com/ societywork/sciencenature/Doctor-Assisted_Suicide.asp); S. Bernstein, *Compassionate murder* (at: http://aish.com/societywork/sciencenature/Compassionate_Murder.asp); D. Eisenberg (1999), *End of life choices in Halacha* (at: http://www.jlaw.com/Articles/ EndofLife.html).

32. There are three exceptions to this: the Commandments concerning idolatry, murder and prohibited relations.

33. Judaism has generally taken the position that to be *in God's image* refers to the fact that human beings, unlike animals, have the ability to reason, to know good from evil, and to make moral choices. On the other hand, the wide variety between humans is said to be proof of God's greatness, given that each person is unique–not identical, not coming from the same mould–despite the fact that we all came from Adam. See Telushkin (1991), p. 529.

34. Rabbi Shraga Simmons, *Siamese Twins*, at: (http://aish.com/societywork/ sciencenature/Siamese_Twins.asp).

35. See H. S. Kushner, *Living a life that matters*, London: Sidgwick & Jackson, 2001, pp. 52-53.

36. See David L. Freeman & Judith Z. Abrams, *Illness and health in the Jewish tradition*, Philadelphia: Jewish Publication Society, 1999.

37. Morton Siegel comments: "Further, the tradition holds that the individual with a disability represents an individuated need. This person is not a reflection of invidious progenitors. His or her disability is not the result of theodicy. It is not an affliction, nor the baneful result of transgression on the part of the parents; nor is it a matter of 'sin.' What has happened, in the technical usage of the term 'natural,' is a physiological or psychological development which is non-valuational. While the individual, accordingly, is the concern of the family, s/he is not the 'black sheep' of the family. S/he is not the albatross perched on the family tree. Today, of course, such an observation is quite gratuitous (or should be). It was much less so in ancient days" (in *Seminal Jewish Attitudes Toward the Handicapped*, at: http://www.rac.org/issues/issuedr.html).

38. *Rabbi Perl On-line*, at: (http://www.rabbiperl.com/issues/iss9.htm).

39. *Rabbi Perl On-line*, ibid.

40. *Rabbi Perl On-line*, ibid.

41. M. K. Siegel, *Seminal Jewish attitudes toward the handicapped*, at: (http://www. rac.org/issues/issuedr.html).

42. The S. Daniel Abraham & Ira L. Rennert Torah Ethics Project & The Lili And William Goldberg Resource Library for Ethical Education, Sources & questions for the whole family, at: (http://www.orthodoxcaucus.org/ads/ad13.htm).

43. See Note 12 (above)

44. Morton K. Siegel, *Seminal Jewish attitudes toward the handicapped,* at: (http://www.rac.org/issues/issuedr.html).

45. Tova, meaning good, is not the true name of the child (as she was at the time). This is otherwise based on a true experience.

46. Gerald Weider, *Living up to Torah*, at: (http://uahc.org/torah/issue/990418.shtml).

47. M. K. Siegel, op. cit.

48. Interestingly, Telushkin (2000) writes that the most common application of this principle is in the area of giving advice: "When a person seeks advice, he has a right to expect that the guidance being offered is intended solely for his benefit. If, for some reason, a person feels incapable of offering neutral advice, he is obligated to explain why or to offer no advice at all" (p. 158).

49. See J. Telushkin, *The book of Jewish values*, New York: Bell Tower, 2000, pp. 44-47.

50. Although Maimonides, Rabbi Moshe ben Maimon, also known as Rambam, wrote *Mishneh Torah* (Review of the Torah) in the 1180s, it is still considered to be authoritative on almost every conceivable topic of Jewish law. His views on Tzedakah (Mishne Torah 7:7) are well known. Among other places, they can be found in *Hilchot Matnot Ani'im–Presents for the poor*, 10th chapter, 10th Halacha, as cited by Zvi Roth at: (http://rambam.cjb.net/).

51. *Rabbi Perl On-line*, op. cit.

52. *Rabbi Perl On-line*, op. cit.

53. *Rabbi Perl On-line*, op. cit.

54. While Jews are often described as a race, this term brings with it many complexities which are unimportant for current purposes.

55. My view on genetic research is that (a) genetic research will never solve the problem of disability because most disabilities do not have a genetic base, and (b) the huge investment in genetic research is based on economic rather than human values. Dealing with the problem of 'drink-driving' could have a greater impact on the incidence of disability than any findings relating to the human genome. Ensuring access to clean water and basic health care, removing landmines and preventing war are serious ways of drastically reducing the disabled population.

56. D. Gordis, *God was not in the fire*, Touchstone Books, New York, 1995, p. 187, cited by P. *Nadel* in *Acting with God in mind*, at: (http://uahc.org/torah/issue/990418.shtml).

REFERENCES

Abraham, A. S. (1996). *The comprehensive guide to medical Halachah* (2nd edition), Jerusalem: Feldheim.

Abrams, Judith Z. (1998). *Judaism and disability: Portrayals in ancient texts from the Tanach through the Bavli*, Washington DC: Gallaudet University Press.

Basser, L. A., & Jones, M. (forthcoming). The *Disability Discrimination Act*: A three dimensional approach to operationalizing human rights. *Melbourne University Law Review*.

Bernstein, S. *Compassionate murder*. Retrieved from: http://aish.com/societywork/sciencenature/Compassionate_Murder.asp

Bernstein, S. (2001). *Doctor-assisted suicide*. Retrieved from: http://aish.com/societywork/sciencenature/Doctor-Assisted_Suicide.asp

Cantor, A. (1995). *Jewish women Jewish men*. San Francisco: Harper.

Chenoweth, L. (1999). A long road to justice: Sexual abuse of people with disabilities. In M. Jones & L. A. B. Marks (Eds.), *Disability, divers-ability and legal change*. Dordrecht: Martinus Nijhoff.

Cook, S., & Slee, R. (1999). Struggling with the fabric of disablement: Picking up the threads of the law and education. In M. Jones, & L. A. B. Marks (Eds.), *Disability, divers-ability and legal change*, Dordrecht: Martinus Nijhoff.

Deutsch, H., & Nussbaum, F. (Eds.) (2000). *'Defects': Engendering the modern body*. Ann Arbor: University of Michigan Press.

Fitzgerald, J. (1999). Bioethics, disability and death: Uncovering cultural bias in the euthanasia debate. In M. Jones, & L. A. B. Marks (Eds.), *Disability, divers-ability and legal change*. Dordrecht: Martinus Nijhoff.

Freeman, D. L., & Abrams, J. Z. (1999). *Illness and health in the Jewish tradition*. Philadelphia: Jewish Publication Society.

Greenberg, B. (1981). *On women and Judaism*. Philadelphia: Jewish Publication Society of America.

Hertz, J. H. (Ed.) (1977). *The Pentateuch and Haftorahs*. London: Soncino Press.

Johnson, K. (2002). The pied piper plays again . . . The lure of contractualism. In T. Carney, & A. Yeatman, *The new contractualism*. Sydney: Federation Press.

Jones, M., & Marks, L. A. B. (2000). A bright new era of equality, independence, and freedom—Casting an Australian gaze on the ADA. In L. Francis, & A. Silvers (Eds.), *Americans with disabilities*. Routledge.

Jones, M., & Marks, L. A. B. (forthcoming). Fostering inclusive societal values through law. *International Journal of Children's Rights.*

Jones, M., & Marks, L. A. B. (2001). Law and people with disabilities. *International Encyclopaedia of the Social and Behavioural Sciences.* Title 3.8.133; Discipline: Law.

Jones, M., & Marks L. A. B. (1999). Law and the social construction of disability. In M. Jones, & L. A. B. Marks (Eds.), *Disability, divers-ability and legal change.* Dordrecht: Martinus Nijhoff.

Jones, M., & Marks, L. A. B. (1994). The dynamic developmental model of emerging rights in children. *International Journal of Children's Rights, vol. 2,* pp. 265-291.

Jones, M., & Marks, L. A. B. (2000). Valuing people through law: Whatever happened to Marion. In M. Jones, & L. A. B. Marks (Eds.) *Explorations on Law and Disability in Australia,* Special Issue of *Law in Context.* Sydney: Federation Press, pp. 147-181.

Kaplan, A. (1998). The infinite light. In *The Aryeh Kaplan anthology 1.* NCSY.

Kolatch, Alfred J. (1985). *The second Jewish book of why.* New York: Jonathon David Publishers.

Kushner, H. S. (2001). *Living a life that matters.* London: Sidgwick & Jackson.

Maguire v Sydney Organising Committee for the Olympic Games [2000], EOC 93-041; [2001] EOC 93-124.

Meiselman, M. (1978). *Jewish women in Jewish law.* New York: Ktav Publishing House.

Mitchell, D. T., & Snyder, S. L. (2000). *Narrative prostheis: Disability and the dependencies of discourse.* Ann Arbor: University of Michigan Press.

Rabbi Perl On-Line. At http://www.rabbiperl.com/issues/iss9.htm

R. v. Latimer [2001], 1 S.C.R. 3, 2001 SCC 1

Rosner, F. (2001). *Biomedical ethics and Jewish law.* New Jersey: Ktav.

Siegel, M. K. *Seminal Jewish attitudes toward the handicapped.* Retrieved from: http://www.rac.org/issues/issuedr.html

Simmons, S. *Siamese twins.* Retrieved from: http://aish.com/societywork/sciencenature/Siamese_Twins.asp

Soloveitchik, J. (1989). *Man of faith in the modern world, vol. 2.* New Jersey: Ktav Publishing.

Telushkin, J. (1991). *Jewish literacy. New York:* William Morrow & Co.

Telushkin, J. (2000). *The book of Jewish values.* New York: Bell Tower.

The S. Daniel Abraham & Ira L. Rennert Torah Ethics Project & The Lili and William Goldberg Resource Library For Ethical Education. Sources and questions for the whole family. Retrieved from: http://www.orthodoxcaucus.org/ads/ad13.htm

Thomson, R. G. (1997). *Extraordinary bodies: Figuring physical disability in American culture and literature.* New York: Columbia University Press.

Umansky, E. M. (1992). Piety, persuasion and friendship: A history of Jewish women's spirituality. In E. M. Umansky, & D. Ashton (Eds.), *Four centuries of women's spirituality.* Boston: Beacon Press.

The Human Connection:
A Case Study of Spirituality and Disability

Pam McGrath, PhD
Christopher Newell, PhD

SUMMARY. This paper utilizes a case study of a woman in the final stage of Frederick's Ataxia, who, together with her carer, participated in an interview just days before she died. As a consequence of impairment associated with the later stage of the disease, the participant's verbal communication was limited. There are various ways in which individuals who are confronting the end of life experience spirituality. For this woman, spirituality was expressed as a connection with significant others, rather than as religiosity. Key findings are expressed in terms of the importance of insights offered by people with non-verbal communication, spirituality rather than religiousness, and the importance of domi-

---

Dr. Pam McGrath is Research Fellow, Centre for Social Science Research, School of Nursing and Health, Central Queensland University, and runs a broad program of psychosocial research on the impact of serious illness.

Address correspondence to: Dr. Pam McGrath, Centre for Social Research, School of Nursing and Health, Central Queensland University, Rockhampton, QLD, 4702, Australia (E-mail: p.mcgrath@cqu.edu.au).

Dr. Christopher Newell is Associate Professor, University of Tasmania's School of Medicine, an Anglican priest, and a person with disability.

Address correspondence to: Dr. Christopher Newell, School of Medicine, University of Tasmania, GPO Box 252-33, Hobart, Tasmania, 7001, Australia (E-mail: Christopher.Newell@utas.edu.au).

[Haworth co-indexing entry note]: "The Human Connection: A Case Study of Spirituality and Disability." McGrath, Pam, and Christopher Newell. Co-published simultaneously in *Journal of Religion, Disability & Health* (The Haworth Pastoral Press, an imprint of The Haworth Press, Inc.) Vol. 8, No. 1/2, 2004, pp. 89-103; and: *Voices in Disability and Spirituality from the Land Down Under: Outback to Outfront* (ed: Christopher Newell, and Andy Calder) The Haworth Pastoral Press, an imprint of The Haworth Press, Inc., 2004, pp. 89-103. Single or multiple copies of this article are available for a fee from The Haworth Document Delivery Service [1-800-HAWORTH, 9:00 a.m. - 5:00 p.m. (EST). E-mail address: docdelivery@haworthpress.com].

ciliary palliative care. The most important gift that pastoral carers, and carers in general, have to offer is the gift of relationship. *[Article copies available for a fee from The Haworth Document Delivery Service: 1-800-HAWORTH. E-mail address: <docdelivery@haworthpress.com> Website: <http://www. HaworthPress.com> © 2004 by The Haworth Press, Inc. All rights reserved.]*

KEYWORDS. Spirituality, disability, chronic illness, palliative care

In this article, we utilize an Australian case study of a person with disability with no particular religious belief, but with a deeply expressed spirituality, to explore some of the important lessons with regard to the human connection found in our daily spirituality. It has been argued by some commentators that Australia is the most secular society in the world. While most members of the Australian population still express some religious adherence, the most rapidly growing statistic over the last few national censuses is that of the number of atheists.

Accordingly, the starting point for our article, and indeed the way in which this case study operates, revolves around the notion of spirituality, rather than religiousness. So what do we mean by this rather slippery term–and state of being–a state which we would suggest is common to the human condition? As Taylor and Ferzt (1990) suggest, "spirituality is defined as that part of the self where the search for meaning takes place" (p. 48). Indeed, as Wald and Bailey (1990) suggest, "spirituality is concerned with the transcendental, inspirational, and existential way to live one's life, as well as, in a fundamental and profound sense, with the person as a human being" (Wald & Bailey, 1990, p. 64).

Yet, perhaps the best definition is found in Sumner's work, including the perceptive recognition of the fundamental differences between religiousness and spirituality:

Spirituality is a basic human phenomenon that helps create meaning in the world. Religion is a specific manifestation of spirituality's drive to create meaning in the world. It can be thought of as part of spirituality, although spirituality is not necessarily related to religion. (Sumner, 1998, p. 26)

The two writers of this article come to this piece of research with markedly different backgrounds. We are united by our very spirituality, as variously defined above; yet we have very different approaches. One of us, McGrath, is a bioethicist who views research as an important instrument for translating insights about the human experience of illness into programs for health care delivery and health policy development, and is thus presently exploring the significance and relevance of the notions of spirituality and spiritual pain. On the other hand, Newell is an Anglican priest and practising ethicist who lives with disability and has a particular interest in the end-of-life and disability issues. For us, it is not just our collegiality and friendship which bind us together but the sense of the sacred that we encounter in the end-of-life work, which means we are drawn together in mystical ways as human beings–ways that are difficult to define. This is particularly manifest in times of trial and adverse circumstances: from war to traumatic death to palliative care settings.

In reviewing the literature, it became apparent that little research has been undertaken regarding the spiritual dimension of the experiences of people with disabling conditions as they near death.

THE RESEARCH

The research project from which this case study is drawn represents the first time substantial funds have been provided by a major Australian medical research organization for work on spirituality. The study, which was funded by the Queensland Cancer Fund for two years, examines the relevance of the notion of spirituality and spiritual pain for hospice patients (Arm A), their carers (Arm B), the health professionals who look after them (Arm C), cancer survivors (Arm D), and patients undergoing curative care in a hospital setting (Arm E). The findings reported in this paper are presented from the arm of the research that explores aspects of spirituality in relation to hospice patients (Arm A).

The participants in this arm of the study are enrolled through the Karuna Hospice Service, a community-based palliative care service in Brisbane. Prospective participants are contacted and told of the study and invited to participate in an interview. Participants are informed of their ethical rights (such as informed consent, confidentiality, and right to withdraw) before they agree to participate, and a written consent is obtained prior to the interview. The University of Queensland Ethics Committee approved the study.

DEMOGRAPHICS

The findings (case study) presented are from one interview with an atypical participant in a target group mainly consisting of people with cancer. The female participant, who we will call Georgina, was 55 years of age and was diagnosed with Frederick's Ataxia at the age of fourteen. By the age of twenty-one her mobility was restricted and required the use of a wheelchair. In the last few years the progression of the disease had been very rapid, and Georgina died not long after the interview. Although Georgina's verbal expression was restricted because of communication impairment associated with the later stages of her disease, it was decided to offer her the opportunity to participate. Too often, research methodologies can silence the voices of those with communication difficulties. Georgina and her carer accepted the invitation and participated willingly and with enthusiasm. While some might focus on the limitations to communication imposed on her because of her disease, we suggest that this case study makes an important contribution because it highlights the various ways, predominantly non-verbal, in which individuals can communicate despite very real communication impairments.

FINDINGS

There are many important findings which arise from exploring Georgina's world:

Constant Non-Verbal Communication Between Carer and Georgina

During the interview the carer sat on a stool in front of Georgina, constantly massaging her feet while maintaining eye contact with both Georgina and the interviewer. The carer displayed an obvious ease and lengthy experience with the physical condition. This was despite the somewhat frightening symptoms of Georgina's disease, such as continually needing to gasp for breath.

Throughout the interview, agreement with what the carer was saying was constantly being reflected in the facial expressions of Georgina, as she laughed, cried, smiled, nodded and in many other non-verbal ways demonstrated unity with and support for the statements made. At times, evidence of the non-verbal communications was reflected in the words of the carer, who always acknowledged such gestures and used such expressions as a medium for including Georgina in the ongoing dialogue. The following excerpts provide some examples of the powerful non-verbal communication recorded during the interview. These demonstrate the overt but silent richness of the communication that characterized the interview.

> "She has done very, very well for herself–very, very independent–she's an inspiration to a lot of other people really. [Tears roll down the face of Georgina, who looks at the carer with gratitude. The degree of empathy is clear.] Don't go teary [carer says to Georgina]."

"We do bits and pieces over the years–eh? [to Georgina]–cook you yummy food . . . [Georgina laughs]."

"She knows that everything is looked after–hey? [to Georgina]–and that is very important to her [Georgina nods enthusiastically]."

"We have an older woman on the crew of carers, and she's like our mum, isn't she? [Georgina laughs]."

At one point in the interview, the non-verbal communication was so dominant that the interviewer raised the issue for discussion and clarification. As the following excerpt shows, the carer's response indicated that such communication was not just a function of her individual relationship with Georgina but was characteristic of the way all of the carers in the team related to Georgina.

Interviewer: You obviously do communicate well. I can see it is as if you are having a conversation even though [Georgina] doesn't . . . respond with words?

Carer: Oh, yes!

Interviewer: So you obviously know each other's thoughts very well?

Carer: Yep, most of us do. It is really hard when you bring on a new carer, because they don't know [Georgina] at all, and they can't understand her talk. It takes about twelve weeks for a new carer to actually understand.

However, the carer did qualify the statement with a reference to her special relationship with Georgina, and said, "I think I cope best out of everyone."

Not Religiosity but Spirituality

It was clearly stated that neither the carer nor Georgina was religious. When asked about the notion of spirituality, the carer indicated that the concept was relevant, and noted that the idea of spirituality was talked about in the network of people caring for Georgina. With the clear statement, "No, I don't find that a difficult word," the carer proceeded to articulate her interpretation of spirituality, with Georgina nodding in agreement. The central notion was that of human interconnection; as the carer succinctly stated, "we are all very connected." There was a sense of 'spiritual pride' expressed both verbally and non-verbally in descriptions of the strong bonds of connection between Georgina and the carers. Because the connection was happening, to a large degree, at an intuitive, non-verbal level, it was perceived and described as a somewhat 'psychic' phenomenon:

> *Carer*: Another of the carers is a very, very psychic person. She knows what [Georgina] wants to say before she even opens her mouth. So, yes, I think we are all pretty well connected to [Georgina] here. She's got a lot of [the] psychic about her own self; that is probably why we are all connected so well.

The All-Consuming Nature of the Disease

When asked by the interviewer to talk about what sense was made of the illness and the illness experience for both the patient and carer, it was stated that particularly during this late stage of the illness, meaning-making centered around the struggle to continue with living in spite of the severe and continuous demands of the illness:

> Well, it just consumed her really. She's sort of coped well–she's coped very well–just starting to get nagging now, for her. I mean, it's very tiring for her and for us, day in and day out, but we've got along.

The stress of coping with such a long-term illness, on the part of the carers, can be seen in the following statements:

> Her health has deteriorated pretty quickly in the last couple of months. But, I mean, everyone here is very well. We put our emotions aside, because [Georgina] gets upset very quickly. So, yes, we just try and cheer her up if she's feeling gloomy and down. She has a lot of pain and she doesn't like to take medication and things all that much; so, we try to help her out without using all the drugs and what-not that she has.

Here we need to recognize that carers bring their own concerns, cares, and perspectives to bear, even in responding on behalf of a client. During such difficult times, leaving the situation to go home does not relieve the stress:

> I mean it is pretty hard going when she is having a bad day. You feel pretty awful when you go home. I don't like going home–I'm thinking, okay, is the next person coming on tomorrow going to look after her?

Such statements reflect the difficult demands of terminal illness as a journey through illness and disability, and these need to be set in the context of reports on earlier "fun times" for Georgina and the team of carers:

We'd come and have chats, go out partying, and that's all slowed down now. We've had our fun times–haven't we [to Georgina]–over those years? Yes, it was a bit of fun. All the carers go–yes, a big group of us get in a big fat taxi and off we'd go . . . probably six months ago would be the last time. She doesn't have the energy or the strength these days to go out much.

Non-Acceptance of the Disease

It was clearly stated that the process of coming to accept the disease and its implication was *not* a dimension of Georgina's illness journey or the meaning she was making from her disease:

Interviewer: Would I be right that you've learnt to live with it over time?

Georgina: [Shakes her head in disagreement and looks to the carer]

Carer: No, she has never accepted it. No, doesn't like the idea of it at all.

Rather than acceptance, the notion that was posited was the capacity to cope with living, in spite of the disease. However, it was noted that at this late stage of the disease, Georgina was beginning to feel "fed up" with the stress of dealing with the demands of her illness:

Carer: The later stages of her illness are really starting to cheese her off. She's fed up–aren't you?

Georgina: [Looks at her with sadness and frustration]

Carer: Very fed up.

The lack of acceptance of the disease was seen as a reason for her refusal to accept appropriate pain management regimes. As can be seen by the following dialogue, for Georgina, pain management signified a submission to a disease that she would never accept. Her independent rejection of pain management was in some ways a symbolic protest against allowing her disease to have the final act of control over her life.

Carer: I know that she's in a great deal of pain. Because she's so stubborn, too, that doesn't help [carer laughs]. As she was told last week, she is taking the pothole road instead of the freeway (laughs). She is slowly coming over to the freeway.

Interviewer: And could you explain that?–[Georgina] could just nod if she agrees with the explanation–why is it important not to take painkillers?

Carer: Yes, I just think it's maybe not totally accepting the disease. Would I be right there? [to Georgina]

Georgina: [Nods in agreement, whilst a tear rolls down her cheek]

The carer then went on to explain that the lack of acceptance was part of Georgina's determination to keep going in spite of the disease.

Carer: Yes, I mean she's just very determined to not let it keep her down, you know. It is like, "Alright, I've got a disease, I'm living with it, but I'll be buggered if I'm going to sit here and let it consume me." You know, that sort of thing. She tries not to think about it.

This lack of acceptance of the disease is an important aspect of Georgina's meaning making, particularly during this terminal stage of the illness trajectory. As a consequence, a non-medical approach to her care is seen as essential to her meaning making, and the opportunity to remain at home is highly valued and significant: "She doesn't like hospitals. We don't call ambulances or go to hospitals; we try to deal with all here. We have a very, very supportive doctor."

The Strength to Keep Going

For Georgina, the strength to cope was not attributed to any religious belief. It was the connection with others, carers and friends, which was reported as the key factor in sustaining Georgina during her life of struggling with the disease:

Carer: She's had a lot of family support, but mainly friends and carers–friends that she's known all her life that still give her their time, really.

Interviewer (to Georgina): Yes, so that is the most important thing. Have you had a religion or theology that gives meaning to this, or not? Or has it just been the connection with other people?

Carer: Yes, connecting with other people.

Interviewer: So, it's not a religion, it's just connecting with people who really care about her?

Carer: Yep!

Georgina was described as having a "very positive outlook on life" that sustained her during her difficult life. Her approach to her illness was to always have a project to do, such as writing a book, and to keep the positive determination to "get on with it."

The carer also indicated that religion was not a factor in her life, and clearly stated that she did not need a religious framework to make sense of her commitment to caring for her friend. For the carer, the sense of meaning she gains from the illness experience is framed in terms of the 'natural' and 'inner' satisfaction she receives from the process of caring and her personal relationship with Georgina:

> *Interviewer* (to carer): And what about yourself, do you have a religion or some framework or personal experience that gives meaning to this?
>
> *Carer*: Oh, yes, I just feel good about doing it. I'm doing it for [Georgina]; she's my mate. Yes, she saw me have all my children, and saw them grow up too fast. Even the kids come here, and rub her hand, and paint her fingernails and stuff like that.

The central principle, or value, informing the relationships between the carers and Georgina was reported to be that of autonomy. The carer indicated that it is essential for Georgina to be in control of what happens in her own home and in relation to her care:

> She is very clean and tidy and very regimented in routine, and if you get someone in here that goes, "Oh that's silly the way she does that," then it is not going to work. It is her way, and so, I mean if we don't agree with her not taking her medication, well, it's her choice and we have to support that choice. . . . It is her life and it's her body.

As spirituality was seen as connection with significant others, rather than religion, it was indicated that the appropriate spiritual response to the situation was to provide support that fostered the network of human connections. Spiritual support was not seen as the provision of pastoral counseling, but, rather, access to appropriate supportive services to allow Georgina to remain at home in the network of significant relationships. The carer indicated that there was a lack of such supportive services, which made the process of caring quite burdensome:

> Government really needs to look now at people who have support packages, and at the resource workers that really need to come and spend time with the people. Because they just don't know what their needs are unless they come here and see what is needed. And everyone is an individ-

ual–they can't just say, okay, disabled is disabled, because every disability is different, and they really need to judge each person differently.

The Desire to Stay at Home

The carer observed, accompanied by affirming nods from Georgina, that "the most important thing, in terms of her meaning in life, was to be in her own environment." It was explained that "she loves her home" and felt in control there with the support of her carer team, and that Georgina had a fear of ambulances and hospitals.

In Praise of Palliative Care Services

The carer spoke of the importance of the support they received from the community-based palliative care service that was caring for them. The service affirmed all aspects of Georgina's meaning-making or spirituality–her struggle with the disease, the importance of her connection with significant others, and the meaningfulness of staying in her own home. The most important aspects of the service were their readiness to come immediately when needed, the information and skill they bring and the sense of personal support they offer.

> Oh, Palliative Care have been absolutely marvelous. They have really helped us out a great deal–taught me a lot. We're really pleased to have them coming. We know we can just ring them; it eases her mind. She was worried about ambulances and things like that; didn't want to go to hospital. So once we got those [at palliative care] involved, they said, "Well, you don't have to go–that is what we're here for."

DISCUSSION

This case study has a significant amount to offer an understanding of the inter-relationships between disability and terminal illness and the central spiritual dimension of life. For some who are religious, it may well be a challenging case-study. However, it is apparent that significant aspects similar to theology are present. For example, the God talk that occurs in theology involves meaning-making, the establishment of sacred space, and the expression of relationship and inter-connectedness. These are all present in this interview.

Certainly, the contemporary pastoral care literature tends to focus on the idea of accompanying our patients on the journey, as opposed to proselytizing. Perhaps the most important gift that pastoral carers–and carers in general–have to offer is the gift of relationship.

We also learn of the importance of non-verbal communication; especially where verbal communication is difficult. In Australia, where historically and presently very little policy attention is paid to people with communication impairments, this is of significant importance with regard to appropriate ways of providing support in palliative care environments. However, it is also apparent that this is important for routine provision of advocacy and other forms of disability support.

Perhaps most significantly, in our experience, it is some of the most vulnerable and least vocal people who can learn a lot from our body language and our unease. The late Bill Williams, an American theologian with diabetes and cystic fibrosis, who subsequently died of these conditions, comments on ministry as the following:

> . . . I've been with people who are not made anxious by my brokenness, and I've seen the difference. It is, in fact, the best definition of ministry I have ever heard; I nearly weeped [sic] when I heard it, it so defined what I needed. Engrave this upon your forehead, if you would wish to do good:
>
> *Ministry Is a Non-Anxious Presence*
>
> You can tell such grace by its care, by its attentive ear, by its pace. When it reaches out to heal you, it is to give relief to you, not itself–and when it prays with you, it lets you declare your own burdens, rather than declaring what it finds burdensome about you . . . (Williams, 1998, pp. 32-33)

Of course, no such language of ministry was used; yet, it is apparent that if theological terminology was appropriate then the carer would be seen to be offering ministry to Georgina.

Further, in Georgina's story we also learn of how, in such deep spiritual relationships, it is not just the carer who has something to give to the patient or client. In analyzing the interviews, it is apparent that people with disabilities and terminally ill patients have something to offer to those who care for them. This has enormous implications for Australian society.

As a 'death and disability' denying society, we tend to view dying and disability as inherently negative. Through the non-verbal communication found in this case study, we encounter the giftedness that those on the margins of society and of life itself have to offer to others. The political and spiritual question is whether or not we are prepared to accept that gift. It is also interesting to observe the emphasis upon autonomy, which largely tends to reflect the Australian focus on autonomy as the pre-eminent value.

However, when we delve into the interview a little bit more, we can encounter some of the other values, virtues, and principles (depending upon the language that we use) which are also represented, although there is not necessarily the language for them in a secular environment. The transcript clearly reflects the importance of notions such as justice, and the very clear attention to beneficence and non-maleficence (doing good and avoiding harm) as ethical principles. Likewise, adherence to such values as truth and the integrity of relationships comes through strongly in the interviews. Yet, we would suggest that in Australian secular society there is one pre-eminent value which rules: that of autonomy.

Indeed, this interview tends to reflect the wider social situation where, from the Enlightenment onwards, we as a society have tended to lose some of the language that was once used regarding ethical concepts. This is in line with MacIntyre's (1981) analysis regarding the need to reclaim such virtues. As David Wells recognizes with regard to Western culture and Christianity:

> In the wider society, during the 18th and 19th century, the classical virtues came under fire from Enlightenment ideology, the Christian virtues in particular came under heavy bombardment, and slowly our language began to change.
>
> These classical virtues had always been thought about in relation to the community in which a person lived. To act justly was not an internal attitude but the practice of what was upright in a context where that moral virtue had been put to the test. When we come into the modern period, and as communities begin to disappear, the virtues come to stand alone, out of the social context in which they had formerly been understood. Thus, as MacIntyre points out, the virtue of honor increasingly comes to be understood in terms of a social status that is not awarded because of moral desert but gained through wealth or birth. When the virtues were thus privatized, when they were disengaged from public life, that life had to be governed, not by morality but by social rules that became etiquette. It was these rules that replaced the virtues, and these rules have now been replaced by governmental regulation and by litigation. (Well, 1998: 15)

We would suggest that this case study also raises important research questions. First, it raises questions about the incidence of spiritual pain. For some this may be associated with the non-acceptance of disease. Our spiritual pain is not necessarily dealt with all that well in the Australian context. This case study helps make clear that perhaps the best way to deal with it is by recognizing spirituality as meaning-making, and providing the human bonds of connection as depicted in Figure 1. This dual focus on the significance of connection and meaning-making as aspects of spiritual pain is affirmed in other findings from the study involving haematology survivors (McGrath, 2002a) and hospice patients diagnosed with cancer (McGrath, 2002b).

One question that was not able to be tackled in this particular case study, but is worthy of further research, is whether religious belief can assist with the acceptance of disease processes and dying, as demonstrated in a previously published case study (McGrath & Newell, 2001). Does religiosity provide particular ways of ameliorating spiritual pain, which spiritual expression by itself does not? One further question raised here that is worthy of further research is whether the acceptance or non-acceptance of disability, as opposed to fighting illness, has any important implications for meaning-making, and indeed, a good death, in the context of a person with disability experiencing palliative care?

CONCLUSION

Perhaps most importantly, in this case study, we encounter the connections between a disabling progressive disease and palliative care. In Australia, care patterns are very much based upon either having a disabling predominantly static condition or having palliative care/terminal illness. This case study shows the importance of models of care which deal with transition, especially when people with deteriorating disability end up facing a variety of challenges living at home. These would appear to be a combination of challenges of both disability and terminal illness.

In Australian society, people with disability and terminal illnesses make meaning in a variety of religious and non-religious ways. Yet it is apparent that spirituality is the common ground. It is clear that meaning, acceptance, and ways of dealing with pain are found in relationships, and that these relationships (verbal and non-verbal) have deep spiritual dimensions which are often not named. Perhaps most importantly, we encounter the importance of human connection–spirituality–in dealing with the issues of disability and terminal illness. In Australian society we are so good at denying the reality of disability and death; yet this case study shows the spiritual wholeness which is to be found when we make the human connection we all seek.

FIGURE 1. Flow Chart of Ideas

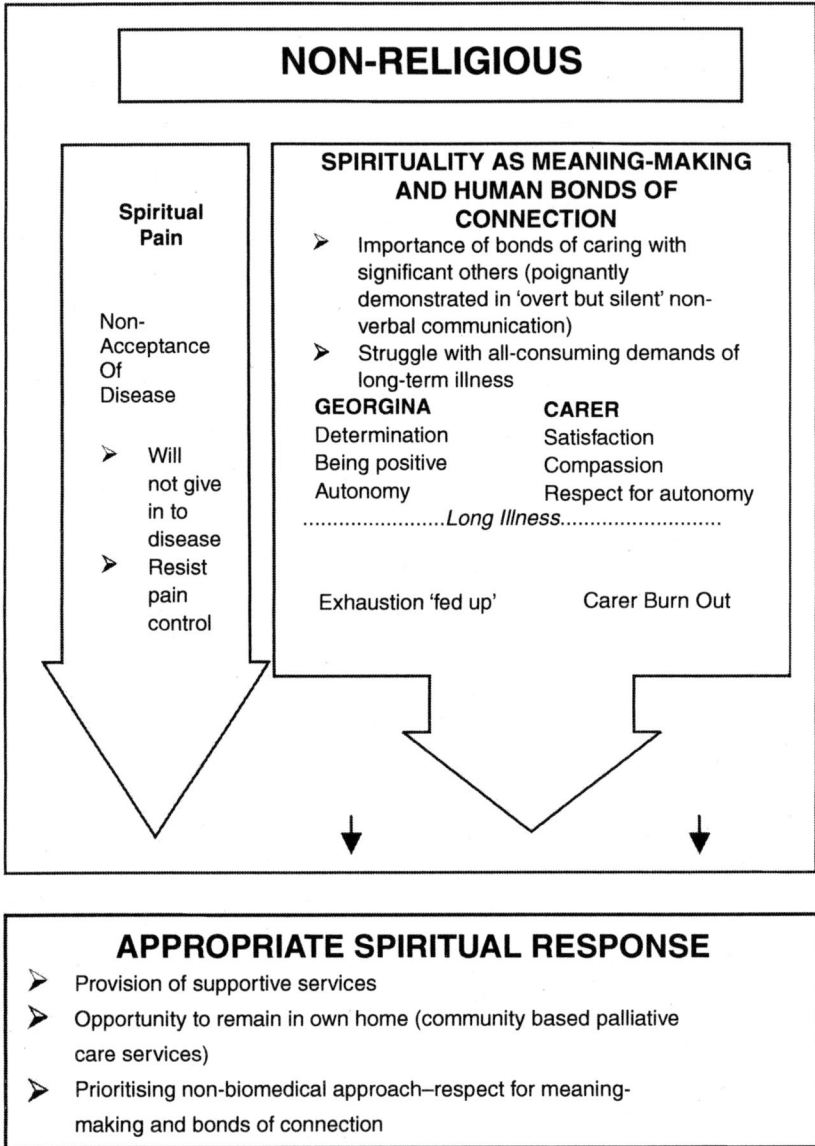

NON-RELIGIOUS

Spiritual Pain

Non-Acceptance Of Disease

➢ Will not give in to disease
➢ Resist pain control

SPIRITUALITY AS MEANING-MAKING AND HUMAN BONDS OF CONNECTION

➢ Importance of bonds of caring with significant others (poignantly demonstrated in 'overt but silent' non-verbal communication)
➢ Struggle with all-consuming demands of long-term illness

GEORGINA
Determination
Being positive
Autonomy

CARER
Satisfaction
Compassion
Respect for autonomy

........................*Long Illness*..........................

Exhaustion 'fed up'   Carer Burn Out

APPROPRIATE SPIRITUAL RESPONSE

➢ Provision of supportive services
➢ Opportunity to remain in own home (community based palliative care services)
➢ Prioritising non-biomedical approach–respect for meaning-making and bonds of connection

REFERENCES

MacIntyre, A. (1981). *After virtue: A study in moral theory*. London: Gerald Duckworth & Co.

McGrath, P., & Newell, C. (2001). Insights on spirituality and serious illness from a patient's perspective, *Interface, 4: 2, pp. 101-109.*

McGrath, P. (2002a). Creating a language for spiritual pain through research: A beginning. *Supportive Care in Cancer*, 10: 8, pp. 637-646.

McGrath, P. (2002b). Spiritual pain: A comparison of findings from survivors and hospice patients. *American Journal of Hospice and Palliative Care*, 20: 1, pp. 1-11.

Sumner, C. (1998). Recognizing and responding to spiritual distress. *American Journal of Nursing, 1*, pp. 26-30.

Taylor P., & Ferszt, B. (1988). When your patient needs spiritual comfort. *Nursing*, 18: 4, pp. 48-49.

Wald, F., & Bailey, S. (1990). Nurturing the spiritual component in care for the terminally ill. *Caring Magazine*, Nov., pp. 64-68.

Wells, D. (1998). *Losing our virtue: Why the church must recover its moral vision*, Grand Rapids: William B. Eerdmans Publishing.

Williams, W. (1998). *Naked before God*. Harrisburg: Morehouse Publishing.

Community Spirit:
Making Space for the Spiritual

Lyn Dowling, MA

SUMMARY. The following paper describes how flexible and relevant pastoral care was introduced into a small school located in a metropolitan area of regional New South Wales. It is a story of both spirituality and community strength and of how these reinforce each other. Introducing the spiritual into our community was an important part of change. *[Article copies available for a fee from The Haworth Document Delivery Service: 1-800-HAWORTH. E-mail address: <docdelivery@haworthpress.com> Website: <http://www.HaworthPress.com> © 2004 by The Haworth Press, Inc. All rights reserved.]*

KEYWORDS. Disability, spirituality, education, children, families, community, social work

According to Swenson, a social justice approach to social work includes economic, political, social, physical, psychosocial *and* spiritual domains, and social work action must focus on ensuring that these domains are available to

Lyn Dowling is a Social Worker and is currently undertaking postgraduate studies (PhD) through the University of Newcastle.

Address correspondence to: Lyn Dowling, P.O. Box 86, Hamilton, NSW, 2303, Australia (E-mail: dowling@hunterlink.net.au).

[Haworth co-indexing entry note]: "Community Spirit: Making Space for the Spiritual." Dowling, Lyn. Co-published simultaneously in *Journal of Religion, Disability & Health* (The Haworth Pastoral Press, an imprint of The Haworth Press, Inc.) Vol. 8, No. 1/2, 2004, pp. 105-114; and: Voices in Disability and Spirituality from the Land Down Under: Outback to Outfront (ed: Christopher Newell, and Andy Calder) The Haworth Pastoral Press, an imprint of The Haworth Press, Inc., 2004, pp. 105-114. Single or multiple copies of this article are available for a fee from The Haworth Document Delivery Service [1-800-HAWORTH, 9:00 a.m. - 5:00 p.m. (EST). E-mail address: docdelivery@haworthpress.com].

Digital Object Identifier: 10.1300/J095v8n01_08

all (1998, p. 527). In the current social, economic, and political context of Australian secular life, spirituality and community strength might be seen to be somewhat out of step in a public school setting. The public school in this story is a 'special' school for children with severe physical disabilities and/or chronic illness. Approximately thirty-five students aged from four years to twenty years attend the school. Building community strength through spirituality (and vice versa) in this setting offers insights about the meaning of disability in our society.

Teachers and teachers' aides working in the school are joined by an assortment of health professionals. In 1996, when the first social worker (the author) was appointed, there were two physiotherapists, an occupational therapist, an occupational therapy aide, two nurses, and a part-time speech pathologist based at the school. The number of health professionals located on site is a reflection of the level of medical need some of the children have. In such a setting, a medical perspective could easily dominate. However, both education and health staff endeavor to integrate their activities; as much as possible, therapy is combined with educational activities. The school is a welcoming place–there is much fun and laughter. Childhood is respected and embraced.

However, because approximately fifty percent of the students have life-threatening or degenerative conditions, the school also experiences times of great sadness. A number of children have died. Families dealing with childhood illness and death have a reputation for being stressed, and distressed. A social work position was established to provide support for students, families, and staff with issues of loss and grief. The decision to appoint a social worker to the school provides an opportunity to reflect on the ways in which children with disabilities and their families are perceived and treated.

In the disability field, professionals and administrators all too often use a *deficits* and *pathology* framework for understanding and intervention. The disability movement has identified the detrimental impact of such a framework on individuals and groups, both in the immediate and long term. Describing this deficits framework variously as the *medical, tragedy, charity,* or *administrative* models of understanding disability, the disability movement proposes, instead, a social model of disability. In this model, disability "is all the things that impose restrictions on disabled people; ranging from individual prejudice to institutional discrimination, from inaccessible public buildings to unusable transport systems; from segregated education to excluding work arrangements, and so on" (Oliver, 1996, p. 33).

An important challenge for the school community was how to apply a social understanding of disability at times of real tragedy, such as the death of a child. A second challenge for the school community was how to make room for the spiritual in what had been considered a secular environment. Our community discovered that these two challenges were connected. Introducing the spiritual into the secular as a regular part of life, assisted us to operate within the social understanding of disability, while respecting individual needs.

I will begin this story at the time of my appointment; although the story itself has a longer history. When I arrived at the school, some of the parents were hesitant about my role on site. Weick and Saleebey (1995) state:

> Families today are under siege as they try to respond to economic, social, and cultural challenges beyond their control. The myths of economic self-sufficiency and psychological normalcy have engendered, in both public policy and family treatment, strategies that isolate, punish, and pathologize families. (p. 141)

If such is the case for families in general, the writings of Michael Oliver (1996) and others would suggest that families living with disability are likely to be seen as even more deficient, problematic, abnormal, or sick. In Australia, social workers and others involved in issues of child protection and income security are often known, rather cynically, as 'the welfare.' Negative encounters with 'the welfare' are likely to occur more frequently for families living with disability, because they often have to interact with a plethora of authorities as they try to access appropriate equipment and support services. Each of these authorities or agencies has particular eligibility criteria; therefore, a multitude of forms must be filled out for assessment and prioritization purposes. In the process, families can begin to feel like public property. The welfare system is not generally viewed by families as supportive; hence, some of the families were wary of my role within this system.

However, educational and health staff were more enthusiastic in welcoming me on site. Some staff sought me out individually, describing how disturbed they were about the deaths of previous students. Because of the high level of distress still exhibited, I thought at first that a particular student had died recently and suddenly on site. In fact, this death had occurred some considerable time ago. The student had left school for the six months prior to his death, and it had not been sudden or unexpected in the way that people were intimating. In this account, it was not the continuing grief, or 'missing the person' that was of concern, but the continuing high levels of anxiety and agitation about the incident. It was about this that individuals came to see me. Some of the staff said that their emotional distress was impacting on how they were dealing with the possible deaths of other students. This was of concern, as it was likely to create particular difficulties for current students whose health was degenerating rapidly.

Paradoxically, the staff as a group often gave the impression that they were, and that we would all continue to be, extremely happy. Publicly, it appeared that nothing nasty or distressing had ever happened, and nothing nasty or distressing was ever going to happen. Clearly, this wasn't quite true, but we seemed to have adopted a 'happiness' culture. I suspect that this culture was partly aimed at protecting the children, and ourselves, from sad feelings. It also seemed to reflect wider cultural messages about how people in general should respond to grief and loss.

Crotty (1998) notes that even though cultures may be *enabling*, they can also be *disabling*. Although there was a strong school culture that interpreted disability from a social model perspective, we had also absorbed other cultural messages about appropriate ways to deal with grief and loss. These messages camouflaged some of the ways in which we might be failing to operate within the social model framework.

However, I think that, at our school, the tendency to deny genuine feelings and replace them with a public parade of other feelings can also be linked to the disabling dynamics of the charity model described by Oliver (1996). The ongoing reality for our little community is that in order to get appropriate equipment–such as electric wheelchairs for the children, or even smaller items–families and staff must do a lot of begging. Begging appears to involve being both *worthy* and *grateful*, and this seems to require *happiness*. We all know this scene. Even with donations in relation to just one child, it can be expected that the children as a group assemble before donors, or before the media, looking suitably cute and cheerful. It seemed that happiness had become our public face, whether or not we were dealing with issues of loss and mourning.

The charity model identifies the ways in which people with disabilities are expected to behave appropriately. In the school setting, I believe that we, the staff, were also conforming to this expectation. A theme I continue to think about is how the dynamics of the charity and tragedy models interact to require reverse displays of happiness and sadness. When happiness should be allowed, a tragedy response seems to be expected; when tragedy elicits true grief, happiness is required. That we as staff seemed to feel we had to collude and participate in camouflaging genuine feelings appeared to me to be significant.

I believe that it is important that we do explore these disabling dynamics and their impact on staff and volunteers further, because:

1. Processes of *disablism* are also damaging for people who work in the disability field.

2. The experiences of workers can have negative repercussions for the people they work with; particularly if these workers or volunteers do not recognize that they are experiencing disablism in action. This may alter the dynamics of their personal and professional relationships with people with disabilities. It may also affect the manner in which they undertake advocacy.

I believe that the impact of disablism on staff and volunteers in the disability literature is ignored; it can inadvertently reinforce an 'us-or-them' dynamic, which camouflages commonalities of experience and the potential for stronger alliance.

One particular event that was graphically described by a number of staff members was the arrival on site of an external team to engage in grief support. This was an experience that people actually were prepared to talk about openly. The eagerness of staff to share this story, and the consistency of the telling, authenticated for me that this was how they experienced it. There was a consensus of opinion that the incident had been significant and personally shocking for them. With each communal sharing of the story, it also became my story and part of my history.

All narratives are interpretations, and, as such, the story might not mirror events exactly as they occurred. It is a meaningful story rather than a factual account of the day. Unfortunately, it does not capture the real support or assistance genuinely offered by the external workers, following a critical incident. However, it is an important story, because what the incident stimulated for the school community was a search for a pro-active rather than a reactive response to critical incidents. The story as it was told to me:

> The crisis team stormed onto the site. These people were strangers who didn't know the children. They took over the classrooms. They couldn't communicate with the children. The children were expected to participate in grief and loss activities with people they did not know. These strangers did not understand or accommodate children's individual impairments. The children were bewildered by the activities and by the strangers. The strangers did not check with the staff or the children about what their real needs were.

Some staff said that they felt emotionally assaulted, both personally and on behalf of the children. With each excited and indignant telling of this story, I even began to imagine a swat team wearing uniforms and boots, jumping off a bus and running onto the site, shouting out commands.

With the best of intentions, our school appeared to have been delivered a crisis intervention, when what people were probably experiencing was normal grief. The system's response appeared to stem from a deficits approach. Saleebey (1996) suggests that a more appropriate response is to look to strengths and resources that already exist within individuals and within communities.

Staff and families began to look at what we could do as a community. We decided that we needed to establish clear protocols that could give us a sense of direction in times of crisis. Individuals needed to feel secure about 'who would do what' and 'what would happen next.' We needed to have some rehearsal of these roles and we needed to know that we could access some ready and familiar support.

We also needed to be genuine about feelings, but, at the same time, accepting of difference. We decided that balancing the control of our own feelings with the needs of the children might indeed mean putting some emotions and behaviors on hold, but we did not need to be dishonest about our real feelings or perform false ones. We needed honesty for ourselves, but we also needed to be able to model this for the children. We hoped that this modeling would serve the children well when they encountered the disabling dynamics of charity and tragedy models across other areas of living. Importantly, we realized that we needed to include a place for spirituality, for ritual, and for the acknowledgement of grief. Activities needed to be open, flexible, and age-appropriate.

As a community, we began to write the protocols. In a crisis, the 'who does what' and the 'emergency number to ring' become lifelines when your hand is shaking and your mind is numb. We did the practical things like contacting the ambulance service to make sure they knew about our potential needs. We made links to other health counselors, and they visited the school in non-crisis times. This allowed staff and students a chance to get to know (and assess) them, and these visitors had a chance to get to know us as people first, before meeting us in a crisis situation. We felt that having a number of familiar professionals, including males and females, offered children and adults a choice of people they could turn to.

We also knew that we needed to talk about grief and loss, and bring it out into the open. We realized that in constantly denying its existence, we had actually ensured that it was always there. Often health interventions around grief and loss are restricted to the secular; we introduced the spiritual.

Sister Annie Laurie of the Sisters of St. Joseph at Lochinvar, who is involved with a community organization called Make Today Count,[1] ran a series of workshops on grief and loss, for families and staff. During these workshops, we examined theories of grief and bereavement in relation to our lived reality. Space was made for personal reflection; space was made for the spiritual as well as the secular.

We purchased books and resources on grief and loss, for both adults and children. We began creating future memories with our photo albums, and we introduced rituals such as memorial services. By using informal occasions (for example, a Mothers Day activity), we were able to re-visit missed windows of opportunity. We became more sensitive and flexible about finding ways to cater for people having to be in different places at different times.

Annie taught us to think about giving people choices and to find creative ways to support them with their choices. For example, when we made a special memorial garden, the children could choose whether or not they wanted to come to a planting ceremony. They didn't have to play in that place in the garden, but it was always there if they wanted to. We were trying to find ways which recognized that children grieve "but they grieve as children, usually not in a sustained way but in spurts on and off during the day" (Lee, 2000). We came to believe that demonstrating a continued valuing of children who have died gives special comfort to those children with life-threatening illnesses.

Annie's spiritual role was specifically written into our protocols, and she made herself available for children, families (including siblings) and staff, at the hospital, in the home, and at the school. This availability extends well beyond office hours. In her wisdom, she became a regular school visitor who just 'hung about' in the playground from time to time–and taught all the children to be naughty! This was indeed great fun for them, and a lesson for us all. Children with physical disabilities who need a great deal of personal assistance are often chronically shadowed by an adult. Laura Middleton reminds us that "children live in the present . . . and that the pleasure of childhood itself should not be lost" (1999, p. 121). It's very difficult to be naughty when there is always an adult watching; yet, surely innocent naughtiness is one of the rights of childhood. Annie modeled for us that when we embrace the moments as they really are, we can enrich our lives. Paradoxically, by acknowledging sorrow, we were better able to celebrate joy.

That year, three children died, and we were very proud that the school community coped. The children were given relevant information about the deaths, by people they knew, and who were close to them. Annie conducted services on site, and the children were able to sing, present their letters and poems, cry and laugh in a familiar presence.

Annie is the greatest. She lives in a house in the community; it is always open to many groups, but every Monday night she hosts some of the students. While their parents might see this as a respite, the children simply see it as "the best time." They play cards, eat what they like, listen to music, and watch videos.

Children with physical disabilities are very often isolated from other children. Large equipment, lack of access in the community, school taxis that come home around dinner time, often combine to insure that the children don't have a chance to mix with other children–to play, to bounce ideas off one another, or to solve the world's problems as a group. While inclusion is great, it is also nice to be able to link up with other children with disabilities: something that can be quite difficult in our great Australian sprawl. Annie's house offers a place where children can play, but where they can also pick their moments to discuss serious issues important to them: issues of illness and disability, of life and death, and of spirituality. And there, they are allowed to be children. Nobody expects them to look grateful, look cute, or to be permanently happy.

Annie has helped us foster resilience. Saleebey states that "resilience is not the blithe denial of difficult life experiences, pains, and scars; it is, rather, the ability to go on in spite of these" (1996, p. 299). By building on strengths, including our spiritual strengths, we as a community feel a lot easier about the hard things in life.

We've also been taught to have lots of fun around Annie. She taught us that when we are confronted with an apparently hopeless situation and a fate that can't be changed, we can change ourselves; especially our way of thinking. We discovered that although we can't choose how or when we're going to die, we can choose how we're going to live.

In our secular society, it appears easy for health professionals to forget the spiritual aspects of grief as we work with individuals or families. We also tend to forget that interventions must be offered flexibly, so that individuals, especially children, can pick their own moments. There are non-clinical ways that we can assist this process. When Annie sits in the playground she can wear any hat, and the children might just as well ask her to play a game of UNO as talk about their fear of having the "same disease as Mary had."

We have had wonderful backup from familiar health counselors for times of crisis, and we have indeed used them for debriefing sessions. But because she offers the spiritual as well as the secular, it has been to Annie that children and families have most often turned.

In our society, individualized or medical models dominate responses to both grief and disability. In these models there is a tendency for staff to think that they have to distance themselves and remain professional. Annie was able to break those barriers down. In particular, one of the things those first workshops allowed us to do was to shed our 'professional' cloaks and join together with families in simply being human.

Because of concerns about inadvertently reinforcing the tragedy model of disability (Oliver, 1996), it is difficult to talk publicly about grief and loss in association with disability. However, I believe that if we are unable to acknowledge that grief is indeed a normal part of life (Dowling & Dow, 2000), we are in danger of reinforcing the oppressive charity model in its place.

Furthermore, if we are unable to discuss grief and loss, we remain unavailable for families and young people, to hear them talk about the other types of grief and loss. These are natural feelings that arise in response to the many attitudinal, economic, and physical barriers that exclude them from the wider community, which I call *structural* grief. As our community discovered, grief that is denied lingers. As staff, we found that children and families deal with life and death issues with great courage and grace. What can be more difficult and demoralizing is the unacknowledged and unresolved grief associated with the structural barriers linked to disability. From a social-work perspective, I found it extremely important to work with families in identifying this structural grief, separating it from other losses, and acknowledging it as a valid grief.

Identifying and naming the structural issues as oppressive and painful seems to free emotional space for families to deal with important personal and spiritual issues. In relation to social exclusion, acknowledging structural grief appears to move individuals towards a social understanding of disability. This understanding then helps provide children and families with a social suit of armor. Introducing the spiritual into the community began a journey that has helped us to make significant changes. We gained community spirit, and, in the process, our community was extended well beyond the school fence.

NOTE

1. This organization originally offered support to adults with cancer.

REFERENCES

Crotty, M. (1998). The foundations of social research, meaning, and perspective in the research process. St. Leonards: Allen & Unwin.

Dowling, L., & Dow, B. (2000, October). Grief . . . a normal part of life? Supporting staff to support people with disabilities who may be experiencing grief. Paper presented at Beyond "business as usual": Pioneering the possibilities for people with an intellectual disability and their families, the 8th National Joint Conference of the National Council on Intellectual Disability and the Australian Society for the Study of Intellectual Disability, Fremantle, Western Australia.

Lee, M. (2000). What do we say to the children? Australian Association of Social Workers NSW Branch Newsletter, 2, pp. 15-18.

Middleton, L. (1999). Disabled children: Challenging social exclusion. Oxford: Blackwell Science.

Oliver, M. (1996). Understanding disability: From theory to practice. Houndmills: Macmillan.

Saleebey, D. (1996). The strengths perspective in social work practice: Extensions and cautions. *Social Work, 41* (3), pp. 296-304.

Swenson, C. R. (1998). Clinical social work's contribution to a social justice perspective. *Social Work, 43* (6), p. 527.

Weick, A., & Saleebey, D. (1995). Supporting family strengths: Orienting policy and practice toward the 21st century. Families in Society: *The Journal of Contemporary Human Services*, March, pp. 141-149.

Solitary Confinement
in the Forgotten Ministry

Elizabeth Mosely

SUMMARY. Life as a latecomer to disability has opened my eyes to the shortcomings inherent in established church ministries. This is my journey, told in anecdotes and poetry, through the discovery of a forgotten ministry within the Anglican Church in Queensland. *[Article copies available for a fee from The Haworth Document Delivery Service: 1-800-HAWORTH. E-mail address: <docdelivery@haworthpress.com> Website: <http://www.HaworthPress.com> © 2004 by The Haworth Press, Inc. All rights reserved.]*

KEYWORDS. Religion, ministry, disability, spirituality, poetry

Although I am nearing sixty, I am just a Lizzie-come-lately when it comes to disability. It is funny, but when you no longer stand upright you lose credi-

Elizabeth Mosely is a writer, public speaker and, now, artist. She is the author of the book and travelling exhibition, with artist Tarja Ahokas, called *Palette & Pen: A Healing Journey.* She has been published in national and international anthologies, magazines, and journals.

Address correspondence to: Elizabeth Mosely, P.O. Box 10474 Adelaide Street, Brisbane 4000, Australia (E-mail: elizmo@iprimus.com.au).

Poetry by Elizabeth Mosely. Printed with permission.

This paper is based on a presentation made to the Visionary Women Conference held in Brisbane, Queensland, in 1999.

[Haworth co-indexing entry note]: "Solitary Confinement in the Forgotten Ministry." Mosely, Elizabeth. Co-published simultaneously in *Journal of Religion, Disability & Health* (The Haworth Pastoral Press, an imprint of The Haworth Press, Inc.) Vol. 8, No. 1/2, 2004, pp. 115-123; and: *Voices in Disability and Spirituality from the Land Down Under: Outback to Outfront* (ed: Christopher Newell, and Andy Calder) The Haworth Pastoral Press, an imprint of The Haworth Press, Inc., 2004, pp. 115-123. Single or multiple copies of this article are available for a fee from The Haworth Document Delivery Service [1-800-HAWORTH, 9:00 a.m. - 5:00 p.m. (EST). E-mail address: docdelivery@haworthpress.com].

bility. People tend to speak very slowly and very loudly, because everyone knows that someone in a wheelchair is both deaf and dim. I have been in a wheelchair for less than ten years now, so I tend not to accept or follow the rules when it comes to society's allotted place for people with a disability–throw in multiple disabilities and you are truly alone.

I also refuse to be silent when I find injustice or intolerance or, worse, indifference towards people who are differently able. To me, those attitudes are more devastating than ignorance, which can be excused. Under the umbrella of the church, even that is not a valid reason for ignoring responsibility to minister to the forgotten not so few.

Churches of other denominations have long-standing organizations for ministry to the disabled; for example, the Little King Movement and Crossroads. However, although there have been attempts to build specialized ministries within the Anglican Church, such as the Anglicare Report, *A Place to Belong: Building Welcoming Communities,* the general perception is that they are dependent on individuals and cannot be sustained beyond personal levels.

An article I wrote, calling for better wheelchair access in our churches, was published in the local Anglican diocesan newspaper. It disappeared into obscurity–people would rather not face unpalatable truths.

I have invited other people with disabilities to come with me to an Anglican church. Without exception, the response to my invitation is: *What is the use? They do not want us. It is tokenism and we are just an embarrassment. They cannot cope with the way we look/talk/act, and then feel guilty about it.* I happen to disagree with that opinion, and feel very strongly that I have a need to be vocal, and to believe that *you* have a need for me to be vocal, as a representative of a neglected segment of the church.

Do not forget that Jesus taught in parables so that the masses could understand Him. He also invariably asked for the sick and lame to be brought before him for healing before teaching commenced. Why is that recognition invalid in today's church community?

Not so long ago a priest placed his hand on my head and asked me, "How do you think you would cope if you were healed?" I replied, "I already am." To me, healing doesn't necessarily mean curing; to me, healing is of the spirit. If you have inner peace, you can cope with anything life throws at you.

There is a great fear of change–any change. I used to travel three kilometers on my scooter to attend my parish church, and yet I had not seen a service in more than four years. I had to park in the aisle of the side chapel; then there were two wheelchairs, so I ended up behind the organ as well.

My poem, "Solitary Confinement," expresses my hurt at being kept apart:

The welcome is warm
the smiles sincere
the Service refreshing
and comfortably familiar
one family in faith;
yet still I sit

in isolation
flotsam, caught by pillar and pew.

Hands reach out in salutation
the unifying grace of the greeting of peace.

Lumped together
like dreaded parasites
segregated stalls
along the wall;
wheelchaired patrons at a theatre,
watchers, non-participants

invisible;
crows seated on a barbed-wire fence.

Denied the pleasure of sharing joy
appreciation tempered by frustration.

The insidious slide
from independence
to societal enigma;
fear and embarrassment
a potent brew;
forgotten by this frenetic world

an aberration
–yet a sword of Damocles;

slowly, inexorably becoming a loner;
a lifelong sentence of solitary confinement.

Like the crow, I know that I can sometimes flap my wings and let out a rau-
cous squawk at an inappropriate time. Like the crow, I can earn a *tutt* of disap-
proval, and my singing voice leaves a lot to be desired, these days. However,
in my head and in my heart, they sound perfect.

I sang with a voice
  so sweet and true;
A soloist free and proud
  to share God's gift
And sing His praise
  with casual joyful Grace.

With sudden force
and grim portent
My voice was taken from me
  in life's discordant way;
Yet I acquiesced inevitably
  to melodic, forgiving balm;

And now I sing with joyful soul,
  I sing within my heart:
and it is sweet and true.

The problem was that I had not shared my feelings with anyone. I am happy to say that finally one of the empty pews was removed so that we could fit in, and the amazing thing is that everyone welcomed the new arrangement. This caught me by surprise, and I was left wondering why. The answer is that the lines of communication had become so blocked by personal prejudice (mine–that dreaded 'them and us' syndrome) and personal insularity (theirs) that no-one even realized that I felt I was not part of the congregation.

The genuine pleasure and support for the changes made me realize the importance of frank and open interaction between members of a congregation. It was a very important lesson for me. However, the isolation still exists in that so far nobody has shared the sacrament with me where I wait before the steps in the nave.

It is a sad fact that very few of our churches are accessible by wheelchair. Ramps were denied, with the excuses of heritage listing and aesthetics–*But it looks so awful!; Who'd come anyway?; It wouldn't be worth the expense*; or even, *They're better off with their own kind.* Their own kind should be human-kind.

The reality is that many 'normal' people in the community appreciate the convenience a ramp provides: the visually impaired, the young mother with stroller and toddler in tow, or the older members of the community. Yet for people like me, most of the churches are no longer open. Freedom to choose my place of worship has been taken from me.

I have not lost my spirituality, simply my ability to walk. The very process of aging causes an ever-increasing number of problems with access for a regrettably large number of people. And these people have often given a lifetime of service to their church and their faith. One day they are there in their usual pew, and the next, they have had to accept the unpalatable reality that they no longer have the right to worship with others. That perpetual struggle to manage even a few steps has beaten them. Their faith has not diminished either–only their mobility.

With agonizing slowness, the church decision-makers are realizing the importance of the need for change in design. The traditional closed sandstone edifice is beautiful, even awe-inspiring, but, sadly, impractical for these modern times or this sun drenched country. It is echoed in the traditional closed and self-righteous belief that piety belongs only to the whole, the upright and the unblemished, and in ostracism of those less able and 'unpretty.'

My first experience of the new multi-purpose parish buildings was a very moving occasion for me (and my wheelchair), being welcomed not only by the people but also by the building itself.

I could choose an entrance to that church and was able to move freely because there were no barriers–no steps halting my progress from gate to door to chancel; pews spaced out to allow free passage. I was able to share the fellowship beside my friends: a new and liberating experience.

This church was at Mount Tamborine, an idyllic retreat behind Queensland's Gold Coast, facing on to natural rainforest. The simplicity of form and abundance of natural wood and glass allowed the glory of the surrounding bush to create a living cathedral:

> Silent communion
> absorbing stillness
> trees that tower
> a glowing arc;
> a cathedral of light
> and spaciousness
>   and peace
> a uniquely Australian blessing
>
> At one with the bush;
>   in spiritual harmony.

I thank God for that reminder that the Church is not just a building. So many times, the physical interferes with the spiritual; especially in that forgotten ministry to the physically disadvantaged. I have some stories to use as illustrations. They epitomize the frustration that people with disabilities can feel:

1. A dear friend of mine is blind. She no longer goes to church. She relied on memory for continued participation, and then they brought in a new service, and new hymnbooks. In her words, she sat like a stunned mullet, totally isolated throughout the service. A simple aid would have been to tape the new service for her to learn at home. She now prays at home and plays familiar hymns by memory on her piano. I might add that she also plays hymns twice a week at a nursing home, and the oldies love it and her, for turning up so faithfully. She told me a wonderful story about a woman with dementia who was unable to speak coherently, but who suddenly sang a whole verse of *Jesus Loves Me*. That woman died a couple of days later. Like so many nursing homes and care institutions, there is no other form of worship available.

2. A grand gothic cathedral in Brisbane is the only one under construction in the world, and we are always being asked to donate to the Cathedral fund, which needs many millions of dollars to finish this fine building. One 'Cathedral Week' when a member of the church hierarchy was being interviewed for the television news, he looked into the cameras and said, 'Our cathedral is open to *all* people.' To tell you the truth, I wanted to throw a slipper at the TV screen. Yes, the cathedral is open to all; provided you are not in a wheelchair. I can get in a side door, but then there is no space for me.

There was the time I visited the Cathedral for a baroque music concert, when another woman in a scooter and I had the choice of sitting behind a huge pillar or sitting at the back in a passageway, as we had been asked not to block the aisle. A young man in a manual chair politely ignored that request and parked near the front. He did not block the aisle completely–but it would have been wonderful if there had been fifty wheelies looking for space.

Of course I do not know what they would have done with them, or what they would have done at suppertime. You, and you, and you could go through the door on the left to the supper area, a matter of a few meters. We would have to go out through a door to the right, down the steep drive, along the street half a block, up the next steep drive, and then back to join the other guests who would have finished their supper by then–forget the return journey. Would it have been so difficult to have the supper in the right forecourt? The solution at that time was to ask someone to bring us a 'cuppa' in the cathedral–surely that is isolation.

I am afraid they will not get a donation from me. A ramp does not cost millions. I believe people are far more important than edifices, for posterity. God does not need aggrandizement.

3. Nor have I lost my need to interact with my own family. On three occasions I have been denied the opportunity to participate in family wed-

ding celebrations. A few steps can provide an insurmountable barrier. I almost made it to one wedding: I managed to get in the front door but became bogged in the coir matting which was set into a depression in the sandstone flooring. I was tipped over backwards and hauled back outside–not a dignified proceeding.

4. I saw my daughter's wedding on video three month's after the event; yet I had been there in person, tucked behind the pulpit where I could hear but was unable to see or be seen.

5. Someone told me about a man who had suffered a stroke and was unable to walk more than a few steps. He went to church and was forced to use a wheelchair, because it was impossible to get the car close to the entrance. She said, "He was so humiliated, he could walk a little." They both failed to see that the wheelchair is a tool, not a humiliation. Society makes it a humiliation.

My friends and family all ask me why I keep trying to change things. I have no answer except that someone has to. I am trying to change hundreds of years of ostracism–how can I realistically expect to make a difference?

I am not alone in my fight for recognition of the fact that a person with disabilities is human: has feelings, hopes, beliefs, and the need to belong. And yet I am totally alone. I am fighting a battle that cannot be won; yet I must still try.

I do not want to prod the conscience; I want only to prod consciousness. Few have the courage to rock the system; few have the courage to insist on change. Few have the courage to hold out their hand and say, "Come, sit by me." We all know the frustration we feel when we cannot understand someone, but that is a fraction of the frustration they feel, every day of their lives, in every interactive situation. This is something to think about when the niggling fingers of impatience or embarrassment scratch our awareness.

"The Masks We Wear," from my book and exhibition, *Palette & Pen*, which says:

> The confident smile
> the happy face
> the positive comment
> the obvious coping
>   the masks we wear;
> essential trappings
> important tricks
> to reassure those we love

–and a poem by the late Catherine Mason, in a report for the Anglicare Mental Health Project, A Place to Belong, contain striking similarities. I believe she would not mind my quoting part of it:

> Hiding myself
> behind the self I present
> to take away my shame
> the shame of being unacceptable
> and socially irrelevant

Here you have two women with disparate disabilities, yet of one accord in their perception of the need to protect, coupled with the longing for someone to reach out and accept us as we are, without the need for subterfuge.

The concept of family groups within the church, where people of all ages, physical differences, and persuasions are brought together regardless of familial relationship, is an exciting opportunity to develop close community ties that will support and reinforce the Christian values so desperately needed today. I can only pray that its scope can be broadened to include people with physical disabilities.

We have much to offer. Major life changes mean major reassessment of priorities and values. The secular gives way to the intensely spiritual; and a new consciousness of true worth becomes a special gift.

This has been one person's journey, one person's cry for help for the many. If you are willing to take notice of my plea for better church access and participation, please do not be complacent. It has to be a package deal. Access to facilities like toilets, halls, and parking are essential too. Acceptance of the person is part of that deal too; tolerance without patronage is vital:

> I make no apologies
> for wanting inclusion
> the need for a ramp
> the only concession
> to my limitations.
>
> Anticipation dies
> as I wait
> with diminishing hope;
> the sound of footsteps
> that do not come;
> concern for others
> who wait and wonder
> where I am.

Frustration simmers,
boils over;
realisation becomes certainty
someone forgets
    the need for a ramp,

And I face society's closed door.

You will embark on a journey, and, like all journeys, it starts with one step–or one ramp. I am sure that as you travel along this new path you will find unexpected rewards. Opening the doors to welcome people who have been denied the fellowship of God's own house will not be easy. However, sharing their spiritual insights will enrich your lives and bring much joy. My vision for the 21st century is that ours will no longer be the forgotten ministry:

May we. . .
Listen to the Spirit and follow its direction;
Listen to the difference and find tolerance;
Listen to the pain and share its burden;
Listen to the dream and change the world.

Listen to the silence and be still;
Listen to the inner self and find peace;
Listen to the love and rejoice in it.

REFERENCES

Mason, C. (1997). A place to belong: Building welcoming communities, in *Anglicare Report*. Brisbane: Anglicare.

Mosely, E., & Ahokas, T. (1997). *Palette & pen: A healing journey*. Brisbane: Spokespress with Boolarong Press.

Giving and Receiving:
We Enter a Faith Program
Thinking We Are Giving
of Ourselves . . .
We Receive Much More

Leonie Reid

SUMMARY. The Personal Advocacy Service is an organization that recruits volunteers to be companions with people with intellectual disabilities. The advocates assist in helping people become part of their community, including congregations, and the program as a whole is infused with a spiritual dimension. Experiences of advocates, participants, and parents are briefly described. *[Article copies available for a fee from The Haworth Document Delivery Service: 1-800-HAWORTH. E-mail address: <docdelivery@haworthpress.com> Website: <http://www.HaworthPress.com> © 2004 by The Haworth Press, Inc. All rights reserved.]*

KEYWORDS. Religion, disability, personal advocacy

Leonie Reid is Executive Director of Personal Advocacy Service.

Address correspondence to: Leonie Reid, 28 Holdhurst Way, Morley, Western Australia, 6062 (E-mail: pas@starwon.com.au).

[Haworth co-indexing entry note]: "Giving and Receiving: We Enter a Faith Program Thinking We Are Giving of Ourselves . . . We Receive Much More." Reid, Leonie. Co-published simultaneously in *Journal of Religion, Disability & Health* (The Haworth Pastoral Press, an imprint of The Haworth Press, Inc.) Vol. 8, No. 1/2, 2004, pp. 125-128; and: *Voices in Disability and Spirituality from the Land Down Under: Outback to Outfront* (ed: Christopher Newell, and Andy Calder) The Haworth Pastoral Press, an imprint of The Haworth Press, Inc., 2004, pp. 125-128. Single or multiple copies of this article are available for a fee from The Haworth Document Delivery Service [1-800-HAWORTH, 9:00 a.m. - 5:00 p.m. (EST). E-mail address: docdelivery@haworthpress.com].

http://www.haworthpress.com/web/JRDH
© 2004 by The Haworth Press, Inc. All rights reserved.
Digital Object Identifier: 10.1300/J095v8n01_10

The Personal Advocacy Service was officially established in 1989 in response to pleas from parents who were searching for a way in which their children with intellectual disabilities (men and women in many cases) could participate in the sacramental life of the Church. Many of these people with disabilities had been living in institutions for a long time, so they were cut off from the community around them. Others were living at home with their families, but had been made to feel very unwelcome when they tried to attend Mass in the local church. Consequently, they had no way of deepening their desire for a spiritual 'connection' in their lives.

Through the Personal Advocacy program, volunteers are recruited from the parish communities and they are linked on a one-to-one basis with people who have an intellectual disability. Support is provided over an extended period as the two people bond together and a personal relationship develops. Within these relationships each person learns to trust the other, and they are able to experience what faith is all about–they are able to experience what a relationship with God is like. They come to know and understand what it means to love and to be loved, to give and to receive, to forgive and to be forgiven. This is really faith in action!

Volunteer advocates and friends with disabilities come together regularly in small network groups, which are located in six different parish centers in the Archdiocese of Perth, Western Australia. These groups provide a 'safe' environment where participants can try many new and different things. The on-going Personal Advocacy program provides ample time for confidence to grow, and, gradually, each person starts to reach out to form relationships with more and more people in the community, and to participate in various community activities and celebrations. In this way, their experiences of life are broadened and enriched: "I have come so that you may have life, and have it to the full" (John 10:10).

The Personal Advocacy program has been operating for more than ten years now, and there have been many wonderful things happen in that time. As we look back, we can confidently say that we have made a difference in the lives of many, many people. Obviously, the most noticeable changes have occurred for our friends with disabilities, and the examples we could cite are many and varied. However, change does not stop there–it also occurs for the advocates as well. Many of our advocates have said, "I joined this program thinking I could do something for someone else, someone who needed me. Yet I have received far more for myself than I could ever hope to give to my friend."

As advocates and 'friends' join other parishioners at the regular Sunday Masses and venture out more regularly into the wider community, they are actually building more positive attitudes towards people with disabilities. Other people see how relaxed the two are in one another's company, and their own fears and inhibitions are gradually broken down. They begin to notice all the things that our friends with disabilities are able to do. They come to appreciate the fact that our friends have a contribution to make, and that the community as a whole is enriched by their presence.

Where people with intellectual disabilities are welcomed in the community, and where they are included in all that is happening, the experience becomes a positive one for everyone concerned. The sense of joy is not only felt by the people with disabilities but is shared also by their families, their advocates, and the community as a whole.

Fay and Tom Tranter, two of the founding parents, reflect on their experience:

> There have been many times in our lives when we have tried to put ourselves in Genevieve's position and think what it would be like to be totally dependent on others for our needs. Immediately, we are challenged to try to understand what she must have to go through to establish a friendship with someone she can trust, and then make that friendship endure. How difficult this must be when she is unable to communicate in a normal way, in relation to her physical, emotional, and spiritual needs.

> People have moved through Genevieve's life–they have come and then gone again–contact is made and then lost. If she lets someone down, she can't say "sorry," and if someone lets her down, she can't say "I forgive." Her friendships are dependent on another person initiating the friendship, and it can only occur when there is mutual love and trust.

> In Personal Advocacy, that love and trust have been forged by some wonderful, generous people, and that is why we hold the service so dear to our hearts. Genevieve commenced in the program at the invitation of Sister Eileen Casey in 1990. At that time, she was living in Carramar Hostel, Pyrton, because of behavioural problems due to residual brain damage from the effects of encephalitis. Only the two advocates who have befriended her since then could explain the difficulties encountered in establishing their relationship with Genevieve; complicated further by the rather overcrowded and understaffed conditions that existed in the hostel. Fortunately, a move to a Catholic Care community home in 1996 changed that situation.

> As a family, we are indebted to Personal Advocacy because of the many blessings it has brought to Genevieve. The painstaking efforts of Genevieve's advocates and other members of the group in encouraging and supporting her to mix with others socially have been of enormous

benefit in assisting Genevieve. This has helped her to cope with the transition from an institutional setting to the residential setting she now occupies under the supervision of Catholic Care.

The advocacy service has taken the loneliness away, built self-esteem, and provided Genevieve with a personal friend and other friends who obviously care about her and accept that she is one of them. Importantly too, the spiritual dimension that pervades the advocacy program is providing her with opportunities to further share in the sacramental and spiritual life of the Church.

Let There Be Light:
Religion, Philanthropy, and the Origins in Australia of Educational Programs for Children and Youth Who Are Blind or Vision-Impaired

Michael Steer, PhD
Gillian M. Gale, PhD

SUMMARY. This paper focuses on the role of religion and philanthropy in the initiation of educational programs in Australia, for students who were blind or vision-impaired. *[Article copies available for a fee from The Haworth Document Delivery Service: 1-800-HAWORTH. E-mail address: <docdelivery@haworthpress.com> Website: <http://www.HaworthPress.com> © 2004 by The Haworth Press, Inc. All rights reserved.]*

KEYWORDS. Vision impairment, blind, deaf, education, philanthropy, religion, history

Dr. Michael Steer is Senior Lecturer in Vision Impairment, Renwick College, Royal Institute for Deaf and Blind Children, University of Newcastle, NSW, 361-365 North Rocks Road, North Rocks, NSW 2151, Australia (E-mail: Michael.Steer@newcastle.edu.au).

Dr. Gillian M. Gale is Educational Consultant, Royal Victorian Institute for the Blind, Melbourne, Victoria, and is Adjunct Lecturer, Renwick College (E-mail: gilliang@alphalink.com.au).

[Haworth co-indexing entry note]: "Let There Be Light: Religion, Philanthropy, and the Origins in Australia of Educational Programs for Children and Youth Who Are Blind or Vision-Impaired." Steer, Michael, and Gillian M. Gale. Co-published simultaneously in *Journal of Religion, Disability & Health* (The Haworth Pastoral Press, an imprint of The Haworth Press, Inc.) Vol. 8, No. 1/2, 2004, pp. 129-143; and: *Voices in Disability and Spirituality from the Land Down Under: Outback to Outfront* (ed: Christopher Newell, and Andy Calder) The Haworth Pastoral Press, an imprint of The Haworth Press, Inc., 2004, pp. 129-143. Single or multiple copies of this article are available for a fee from The Haworth Document Delivery Service [1-800-HAWORTH, 9:00 a.m. - 5:00 p.m. (EST). E-mail address: docdelivery@haworthpress.com].

INTRODUCTION

European settlement of *Terra Australis*, the Great Southern Land, commenced in 1788 when a British penal colony was established on its eastern coast. From this colony, the nation of Australia was born. A number of reasons contributed to Britain's decision to colonize the new land. Most important was its need to relieve its overcrowded prisons. Further, Australia was of strategic importance to the mother country. It provided a base for the Royal Navy in the southern seas and could be used as an entry to the trading opportunities of the region. All of these factors persuaded Lord Sydney, Secretary of State for Home Affairs, to authorize the colonization. Since many readers will possibly be unfamiliar with Australia, or matters Australian (indeed, Australians quite commonly hold that many in the Northern Hemisphere confuse their homeland with Austria), some of the history of its earliest white settlement follows.

On May 13, 1787 Captain Arthur Phillip, commanding 11 convict ships, left Britain for the new colony. He arrived at Botany Bay on January 18, 1788. However, the colonists eventually settled at Port Jackson, a few kilometers north. The ships landed 1,373 people, including 732 convicts, and the settlement became Sydney.

With the hindsight of 215 years, it seems almost incredible that the British Government of that time, while sending out its convicts and soldiers, initially made no provision of any sort for religious ministration to their spiritual and moral welfare (Barry, 1932). Two days before the expedition sailed, through the urgency of William Wilberforce and the Bishop of London, permission was granted to the Reverend R. Johnson, a volunteer, to join it as Chaplain, but without an emolument of any sort and without any sanction or authority. After six years in the new colony, Reverend Johnson, an Anglican of the time, succeeded in building a small church with his own hands and with his own means. The light that he had sparked was almost entirely extinguished by a militarily governed convict society that was declared by a number of competent observers to be "immoral beyond any known immorality." After only a few years, records indicate that in one particular two-year period there were 400 capital convictions in Sydney's population of some 40,000 souls (Barry, 1932). The living conditions of the convicts in New South Wales, Norfolk Island, and Tasmania were described as "Hell on earth." As an example of the inhumanity endemic to public behavior in the early days of the colony, Alfred Barry, Bishop of Sydney (1884-9), has recorded that the colonists' treatment of Aboriginal Australians at this time was characterized by extraordinary cruelty, violence, and bloodshed. As a further indicator of the times, Cleverley (1971) has pointed out that "the colony's first school mistresses were recruited from a pair of petty thieves" (p. 25).

Back in England, Australia was, as Law (1922) has pointed out, considered little more than a far-flung outpost of Great Britain, and only one of the several targets of its social hygiene policies. Educational developments in the colony's earliest days were greatly influenced by British traditions and practice (Watkins, 1987). It was a tradition in which formal schooling was initially not the prerogative of most of the poor, but was generally classical in focus and was considered to be preparation for the professions rather than the trades. Educational policies and practices were molded (as in 2002) in light of the society of the day, with philanthropy and religion as the basic ingredients of the approach. The Church of England initially assumed responsibility for education in the colony. Governor Macquarie extended this system, so that by 1821 there were between 15 and 20 Church of England supervised schools in the colony. According to Potts (1999), Anglican dominance was soon "challenged by the Roman Catholics and Presbyterians who were determined to preserve their denominations in the face of attempts by the Anglicans to extinguish them" (p. 242). Control of education in the colony was more than a matter of religion for the Irish and Scots, who constituted the membership of these latter denominations. It was closely allied with their need to preserve and develop their respective cultural identities. With regard to initiating the education of the colony's blind children and adults, little if anything constructive occurred from 1787 to the 1860s. The first recorded developments resulted from religious and lay philanthropic initiatives. This brief article will examine the impact of those religious and lay philanthropic beliefs on the initiation in colonial Australia of educational programs for children who were blind or vision-impaired.

Scriptural Incentives

Blindness as a focus for philanthropy does not seem to do particularly well in the Old Testament. It is, as a word, generally used to symbolize a lack of moral and intellectual light (Hunt, 1984). The word is sometimes used in connection with "those who grope in darkness seeking light" (Is. 29:18; 42, 6, 7). This is also sometimes its use in the New Testament (Acts 26:18; John 10:21). It is likely that these sorts of references were among those that kindled the desire on the part of early Australian colonists to help those believed to have been lost in darkness, yet who were deemed by holy writ to be eager to be brought to the metaphorical light.

Further, the Scriptures abound with examples of blindness being used as a tool of affliction by the God of the Old Testament, on those who had offended Him or His chosen people. As examples, the blindness afflicted on the men of Sodom (Gen. 19:11) and upon the Syrian army (2 Kin. 6:18). In the New Testament, both Saul of Tarsus (Acts 9:8) and Elymas (Acts 13:11) are inflicted with blindness as Divine punishment. Indeed, the Scriptures bring us prayers for the deliverance from the scourge of blindness (Ps. 13:3 119.11). However, on the positive side, the New Testament is replete with examples of Christ healing the blind (Matt. 9:27-30; Luke 7:21; Mark 8:22, 10:46; and John 9), and of Christ actually removing blindness (Luke 4:18; John 8:12; 2 Cor. 3:14).

It is likely that examples such as the latter were also the inspiration for early attempts by the Sydney colonists to care for and educate those they would have regarded as among their most overtly afflicted and handicapped. In Australia, as overseas, much of the early work in the education of students with disabilities had, as Kauffman (1980) has pointed out, a heavily religious orientation. One of the major initial motivators in the education of students with sensory disabilities was the need to instruct children in religious matters, and it is likely that the first schools had a strong religious atmosphere (Moores, 1996).

EARLY AUSTRALIAN SPECIAL EDUCATION

In Australia today, responsibility for the provision of schooling is shared among the six states, two territories, and the Commonwealth (federal) Government (Blatch, Nagel, & Cruickshank, 1998). State and territory ministers are responsible for the provision of primary and secondary schooling to all students of school age in their state or territory, including those in the non-government sector. All states and territories have well developed policies and programs based on equity principles that aim at providing quality schooling for all students irrespective of their ability, social background, or geographic location. Most policies relating to the education of students who are blind or vision-impaired support the delivery of programs in the "least restrictive environment," appropriate to each student's needs (New South Wales Department of School Education, 1997). This has resulted in the majority of students who are so disabled receiving their education in their local community school. In the years since initial white settlement, the schooling of students who are blind or vision-impaired has come a long, long way.

The earliest formal attempts at offering schooling to students who were blind and vision-impaired have generally been ascribed to the French. Just three years before the settlement of Sydney by the British, Valentine Haúy established the *Institute Nationale des Jeunes Aveugles* in Paris (Scholl, 1886). To the National Institute's Louis Braille (1809-1854) is owed the genesis of the braille code in the early 1800s. Some 50 years after the establishment of Haúy's National Institute, there were three schools for the blind in the United States, as well as schools in several European countries, including Great Britain, Germany, and Russia. Similar developments in Australia arrived some 20 years later.

Initially, Australia, like Great Britain, had no public education system. There was, as Watkins (1987) has pointed out, no clear demarcation between church and state in the early colonial schools. The development of schools and supports for those who were blind or vision-impaired followed patterns of colonization, with New South Wales and Victoria leading the way. The education of students with vision impairment struggled through this early period of Australian establishment and growth with little or no expert advice and negligible government support. This was an era that provided great scope for public philanthropy and religiously motivated philanthropists.

The remaining sections of this paper deal briefly with the initiation, through religious and philanthropic involvement, of educational programs for students who were blind or vision-impaired in all the Australian states excepting the two Australian territories (Australian Capital Territory and Northern Territory). Educational services for students who are blind or vision-impaired in these jurisdictions appear to have been generated by direct government involvement, with students from both territories having initially sent their students to special schools in Sydney. The rationale for treating the influence of religion and philanthropy on the development of educational services by focusing on each State is that Australia did not become a federated Commonwealth until 1901. Until that time *Terra Australis* consisted of a number of separate autonomous colonies, each with its own government and culture. Several colonies, for example New South Wales, had been founded as penal settlements; others, for example South Australia, by free settlers.

New South Wales

As an aid to overseas readers, New South Wales is located on the east coast of the Australian continent. Sydney is its major city. The state has a population of some 6.5 million (Trewin, 2001), who are known to other Australians as 'New South Welshmen' or, variously, 'Sydneysiders.' It became a British possession in 1770, and, as mentioned above, its first white settlement was in 1788. By 1856 it had an elected Parliament and responsible colonial government. It federated with the other Australian states to form the Commonwealth of Australia in 1901.

In Australia's first colony, in 1860, Thomas Pattison, an educator and deaf himself, became catalyst and co-founder of the first special school for students with sensory disabilities in New South Wales. In that year, he became Superintendent of the Deaf and Dumb Institution of New South Wales, which is today the Royal Institute for Deaf and Blind Children. A relatively large body of philanthropic men, representing churches, government, and business administered the institution. Throughout the foundation period, discussions and many debates were held on the need for education of children with vision impairments. The focus of the debates was whether or not their education should take place within a new special school, or whether they should be educated with hearing-impaired and deaf children. Several of the speeches made at the early public meetings of the new Institution are instructive. For example, the Reverend Dr. Dinsmore Lang stated the following on 1 October 1862:

> Deeply must he feel who was shut out of such enjoyments by the deprivation of hearing. It was still a greater deprivation than the want of sight, and the situation of the sufferers under it deserved the sympathy of their fellow men. (Davidson, 1966, p. 7)

The Reverend George King, foundation President of the Institution, emphasized Christian charity at work in the education of the deaf and blind (Davidson, 1966, p. 8).

At a second public meeting of the Institution, Dinsmore Lang referred to information he had obtained from "statistical writers" on the prevalence of deafness and blindness around the world. This information, he claimed, indicated a fixed proportion from country to country:

> And it was remarkable how equal the proportion was in different countries and at different times. It was only when a country had reached a certain state of progress that efforts were expected on the part of the community for the benefit of those so afflicted from their infancy. It was not in the power of a small community to afford the instruction which those persons required, and it had only been from a comparatively recent period that successful efforts had been made to supply this portion of the human family with the education that their unfortunate circumstances so peculiarly demanded. (Watkins, 1987, p. 133)

Influences from overseas also became evident at this early stage of Australian history, including those derived from the United States. The Reverend Dr. Lang obviously had considerable background on the origins of special schools in France and 'the mother country,' and seems to have been familiar with earlier progress in the United States, having visited it two decades previously. He had visited a special school in the City of New York and claimed that Australian colonial society had reached such a state of development that what had occurred overseas could now be emulated in Sydney (Deaf and Dumb Institution of New South Wales, 1870).

It was finally decided, possibly on economic grounds, to admit students with vision impairments with those who had hearing impairments (Watkins, 1987). In 1869 the first six children with vision impairments were admitted to the renamed New South Wales Deaf, Dumb and Blind Institute (Plowman, 1985). This philanthropic development, far reaching for its time, seems to have set the pattern for early educational services in the other Australian colonies. An instructor, a Mr. Cashmore, himself vision-impaired, was hired to oversee the education of the first six blind children. He resigned in 1874; thereafter, children with vision impairments were taught by the same instructors as those with hearing impairments (Kelley & Gale, 1998).

The New South Wales Institute for Deaf, Dumb, and Blind continued to operate for almost 70 years as the only option for students with vision impairments in the state. Its residential school, at which students with vision impairments and those with hearing impairments were educated together, operated until the mid-1950s (Watkins, 1987). In 1879, a separate institution for adults was established and this later became the Royal Blind Society of New South Wales (Kelley, Gale, & Cruickshank, 1998).

The Catholic system of education for students with vision impairments dates to the establishment of St. Lucy's School for Blind and Partially Sighted Children in 1938 by the Dominican Sisters (Kelley & Gale, 1998). Located at Wahroonga in Sydney, it was initially a residential school for boys and girls who were blind and vision-impaired. It currently operates as a co-educational primary school specializing in blindness and vision impairment. St. Edmund's School for Blind Boys was opened by the Christian Brothers at Wahroonga in 1951. It was a residential secondary school, from which the boys went into the community for various public and religious functions. It currently operates as a co-educational secondary school for students with vision impairments, as well as a number of students with learning difficulties.

In 1962, the New South Wales Department of School Education began integrating secondary students into special units in regular schools (Beckenham, 1969).

Victoria

Located on the southeast coast of the continent, Victoria was, until 1851, part of New South Wales. In 1856, responsible government was conferred by the mother country, and the colony formed its own parliament. With a population today of almost 4.8 million, its state capital is Melbourne. Victoria was the first Australian state to make statutory provisions (in 1901) for the payment of Age Pensions, and generally boasts an enviable history of advanced social policy. It is affectionately known to Australians as the 'gumsucker state.'

The first Australian school solely for children with vision impairments was established in Melbourne. The Victorian Asylum and School for the Blind, now the Royal Victorian Institute for the Blind (RVIB), was founded as "a collective philanthropic effort by a large group composed of clergy, politicians, physicians, businessmen, and women" (Watkins, 1987, p. 138). The school opened in 1866 (Kelley, Gale, & Cruickshank, 1998). Its first staff member was a Miss Jones, a trained teacher who had worked in the Blind Institution in Bristol, England (Watkins, 1987). Its early curriculum included reading, writing, spelling, arithmetic and music, with some vocational training in knitting, sewing, and basket making.

In an unpublished history of the RVIB, McCaskie (1973) attributed the "idea of making a separate institution for the blind" to the Rev. James Mirams (p. 5). He was reputedly leader of the fifteen philanthropists who formed the provisional committee that resolved on 1 May 1866 "that steps be taken to establish an Asylum and School for the Blind" (p. 8).

The school began in 1866 on rented premises, with an enrolment of nine students. By the time the present building was opened, there were twenty-one, and until the mid-1970s, there were between fifty and sixty students at any one time. Most students were boarders throughout the term, while some were weekly boarders. Very few attended on a daily basis (Nuske, 1992). The inscription on the front page of the Asylum and School's first annual report read:

> I will bring the blind by a way they know not; I will lead them in paths that they have not known; I will make darkness light before them, and crooked things straight. These things I will do unto them, and not forsake them. (Isaiah XLII, 16)

> I was eyes to the blind. (Job XXIX, 15)

These texts were continued on each subsequent annual report for the next 29 years (Watkins, 1987), and serve to highlight the thinking behind the establishment of Australia's earliest school for the blind. Like its European ancestors in Paris and London and the pioneer schools of North America, it was born in an atmosphere of religious philanthropy. From Haüy in France, through Rushton in Liverpool, and Gridley-Howe in Boston, the charity school for the blind had arrived in Australia. In 1885, secondary subjects were introduced into the school's curriculum and occasionally 'star' pupils received a tertiary education; although, as Watkins has pointed out, this was not the norm.

As in New South Wales, the available records provide no indication of any survey, even of a limited nature, having been undertaken to ascertain the numbers of blind children in the colony, requiring special school placement (Watkins, 1987).

One of the first books available to the children at the school, when braille was introduced in the early 1870s, was the Protestant Bible. Perhaps because of this, and the influence of the gentle and caring Reverend Moss, who was the superintendent in the 1880s, religion played a large part in the lives of the pupils for many years (Nuske, 1992). Children were taught to say their prayers and, before and after each meal, grace was sung. Protestants and Catholics received separate religious instruction, and each went to their separate services on Sundays. This had an interesting facet during the polio epidemic of 1937, as one of the students stated in reminiscence:

> . . . another part of my schooling was during the polio epidemic which was in 1937 and we were in quarantine. That epidemic went from June until about March or April of the next year, so we were in quarantine from June until December and if you were in the RVIB School you were not allowed out, and no one was allowed in. The only people that were allowed out were the Catholics, they were allowed to go to Mass, but the Protestants weren't allowed to go to church. (Nuske, 1992, p. 8)

Alice McClelland, another student interviewed by Nuske, remembered, with a twinkle in her eye, that around the turn of the century the preachers came to the RVIB:

> The only time we ever saw the boys at all was on the fifth Sunday of the month. We used to have a local preacher come down and conduct services on a Sunday night and on the fifth Sunday in the month nobody came so they used to let us go to church. Of course we were very religious in those days and we were glad to go to church on the fifth Sunday because we could walk home with the boys, you see. (p. 15)

In 1961, the RVIB opened a residential nursery and school. By the end of the 1960s, some secondary students were receiving their education in local public (government) schools, and the residential school was located away from the RVIB main campus. The Victorian Education Department initiated a visiting teacher service in 1973 (Kelley, Gale, & Cruickshank, 1998).

South Australia

South Australia was formed into a British province in 1836. It is geographically vast, with its state capital Adelaide located on the south coast of the continent, and has a population of approximately 1.5 million (Trewin, 2001). Its elective legislative council was established in 1851 and its constitution dates from 1856. The colony differed from its neighbors, as the home of free settlers rather than convicts. South Australians are affectionately known as 'Crow-eaters' to their peers.

Educational services for students in the colony who were blind or vision-impaired can be traced to the work of William Townsend. He was a philanthropist who, in 1872, presented a resolution to the colony's government that it should match any funds raised for the establishment of an asylum for "blind, deaf, and dumb" individuals (Murphy, 1965). The Institute's first students were admitted in 1874.

The program's original focus was vocational training, and it was modeled, in the first 100 years of its existence, on programs offered by Victoria's RVIB. By 1915, the program had become the Townsend School. By 1956, the state's Education Department took responsibility for the students who attended it. In 1974, a visiting teacher service was initiated and based at the school.

Queensland

Queensland, with its state capital Brisbane, and a population of over 3.5 million, is geographically vast. It was initially part of New South Wales, but became a separate colony in 1859. In Australia, Queenslanders are affectionately known as 'Banana-benders.'

Similar to events in other states, initiation of educational services for blind and vision-impaired students in Queensland can be traced to religious and philanthropic activity. In 1883, a Mr. J. W. Tighe was trained, equipped, and sent to Brisbane to conduct home teaching programs in Moon type (a form of embossed script invented by Dr. William Moon of Brighton, England, in 1847 (Steer, 2000). Tighe had been instrumental in establishing a similar sort of service in New Zealand. Together, he and a local ecclesiastic, Bishop Mathew Blagden Hale, founded the Queensland Blind, Deaf, and Dumb Institution. The Institution started initially as a trade school. By 1887, a workshop, office, and manager's residence had been constructed on site (Watkins, 1987).

Bishop Hale was highly influential in the initiation of formal education in the new colony and also in Western Australia. Although the product of private tutoring and a Cambridge education himself (Rich, 1991), he seems not to have been particularly elitist in his intentions. Wilson (1957) has suggested that in this regard Hale was too well aware of his Church's poverty and diminishing influence to want to create a denominational and class-orientated educational system.

Initially, the colony sent its young students to Sydney. However, it became apparent that children suffered from separation from their families, and by 1889, Queensland, mainly through the efforts of Reverend James Stewart, started to plan its own school. It was opened in 1893, and funded from public charity, state funds, and by local churches (Kelley, Gale, & Cruickshank, 1998). By 1931 the Department of Public Instruction had assumed responsibility for the school, and by 1956 had started to integrate students who were blind or vision-impaired into the regular school system (Blatch, 1989).

Tasmania

Abel Janzoon Tasman discovered Van Diemen's Land (Tasmania) in 1642. It became a British settlement in 1803, as a dependency of New South Wales. Responsible government was granted in 1856, and in 1901 the 'Apple Isle' became federated with the other states into the Australian Commonwealth. It is a large island, with a population of approximately half a million, situated off the southeast coast of the continent, with Hobart as its capital. Within Australia, Tasmanians are called 'Taswegians' or 'Apple-islanders.'

Education for students who were blind or vision-impaired commenced in Tasmania in 1887 (Watkins, 1987). Prior to this, children thus impaired were sent to the institutions in New South Wales and Victoria. Because of its proximity to Melbourne, most Tasmanian students attended the RVIB program, with maintenance paid by the Tasmanian Government.

One of the Tasmanian students who attended the Institute in New South Wales was Thomas Mercer. On his return to Tasmania in 1882, local philanthropists in Hobart initiated A Society for the Benefit of the Tasmanian Blind. Mercer was appointed its first itinerant teacher, and conducted a home visiting program for adults. A braille library was established by the Society in Hobart in 1894, and the Braille Writer's Association was established in 1897 (Kelley, Gale, & Cruickshank, 1998).

Tasmania was the first Australian state to place the education of students who were blind or vision-impaired under government control, support, and supervision (Watkins, 1987). It was also the first state to legislate (1905) for the compulsory education of children with vision impairments. In the 1970s Tasmania introduced its first visiting teacher service.

Western Australia

In 1791, Captain George Vancouver, in the *Discovery*, took formal possession, for Britain, of the land about King George Sound on the far west coast of the Australian continent. In 1826, the Government of New South Wales sent

20 convicts and a detachment of soldiers to King George Sound and formed a settlement which they named Frederickstown. In 1829, British naval captains Fremantle and Stirling took formal possession of the territory which has since developed as the state of Western Australia, with its capital, Perth. Western Australians are widely known within Australia as 'Sand-gropers.'

As Pritchard (1997) has pointed out, independent non-government schools in Western Australia have produced, over the past century, a well-established religious ethos. This has been partly based on their religious instruction practices and because the religious education they have offered has been of an holistic quality in which religious influence has been pervasive. The interdenominational ethos that has permeated the independent schools perhaps owes its existence to the work of Bishop Mathew Hale, who in 1858 established the Bishop's School. Further, Pritchard has asserted that a combination of the religious practices of the first colonists, from the foundation of the colony in 1829, with the activities of the Anglican Sunday School and the Methodist class meetings in one of the most remote parts of the continent, were an essential antecedent to promotion of a religious ethos in the colony's early elementary education.

The precise date at which the first educational service to individuals with vision impairments in Western Australia was initiated is unknown (Kelley & Gale, 1998). In 1894, a Mr. Davis traveled to Perth (the colony's capital) from Victoria to conduct home teaching for adults with vision impairments. It appears that from this humble beginning, the West Australian Home Teaching Society developed. In 1896, the colony's government provided a grant to establish the Industrial School for the Blind (Western Australian Council for Special Education, 1978). In 1897, the first official meeting occurred of the management committee for the Victoria Institute and Industrial School for the Blind; so-named to commemorate Queen Victoria's Diamond Jubilee. The school was similar in organization to the school earlier established in Victoria, since its program separated the education of students with hearing impairments from those with vision impairments. This agency served both children and adults, who until 1901 shared the same teachers. The aim of the Institution was to provide primary education for children and pre-vocational training for adults. History does not record the numbers of students who attended the facility.

In 1919, an Amendment to the *Education Act of 1871* (Western Australia) provided for the compulsory school attendance of children with vision impairments. From that time, regular government grants were made to the Institute, and the Amendment included a provision requiring the medical certification of students as vision-impaired, prior to their admission.

CONCLUSION

The period from the anchoring of the First Fleet in Sydney Cove to the middle of the nineteenth century (a period of some 60 years) saw considerable activity in the provision of educational facilities for the colony's children and, on occasion, for the children of Aboriginal Australians (Crawford, 1979). Most of this activity was undertaken by the various churches, heavily supported by government funds (Watkins, 1987). Such a policy had parallels with provisions in England, where government initiatives had first taken the form of subsidized church schools. During the initial years, New South Wales was Australia, and "religion has always played a part in the education provided by New South Wales Government schools" (New South Wales Department of Education, 1983). In fact, the early years saw little or no demarcation between Church and State in a penal colony where freedom of thought, speech, and action were at a minimum. From the very beginning it was accepted, as Turney (1975) has pointed out, that the Church of England had a special prerogative in matters of public education.

History indicates that the development of educational services for Australians with vision impairments followed patterns of colonization, with religious and philanthropic involvement in New South Wales and Victoria leading the way. Special schools (Institutions) and special programs for such students struggled through the early period of establishment and growth (1860-1890), with little or no expert advice and negligible government support. It is of interest that only the Roman Catholic Church became involved in this particular form of pioneering endeavor in Australia.

Initially, although the Church of England had assumed responsibility for education, it did little or nothing about the special schooling needs of children who were blind or vision-impaired. This position was challenged by the Presbyterians and the Roman Catholics, but it was the latter who led the way with regard to meeting the special needs of families with children thus disabled. Their leadership might, through the eyes of those in power, have been perceived as being as much about their attempting to meet their constituents' needs in an attempt at preserving their denomination–in the face of Anglican attempts at extinguishing them–as it was about any other source of motivation.

In support of this proposition, in 1879 the Catholic bishops of Australia realized that large numbers of Catholics were not sending their children to Catholic schools, and issued a joint pastoral letter stating that Catholics must send their children to Catholic schools unless given special dispensation by their parish priest (Potts, 1999). So, while the Catholic Church argued at this time for democracy and pluralism with respect to school choice, the openness did not extend to allowing choice to members of its own flock.

While religion is important in the history of Australian mainstream and special schooling, it appears to have generally been associated with economic and other concerns. The Catholic population, for example, was prepared to bear large financial burdens to maintain and pass on its own distinctive cultural traditions, and it is likely that future research might indicate a strong correlation in early Australia between Catholicism, blindness or significant low vision, and low income.

After World War II, the traditional influences exerted by the Mother Country on Australian education began to wane, and it is likely that influences from the United States started to become stronger at this time. The development of Australian special schools for children and youth who were blind and vision-impaired, according to Watkins (1987), experienced difficulties throughout this formative period, with "corporate management negating strong individual leadership, with executive teachers having experience in the education of the deaf and not the blind" (pp. 219-220). All of this was set against a backdrop characterized by vast distances between population centers both in Australia and abroad.

REFERENCES

Barry, A. (1932). Christianity in Australiasia. In E. Baker (Ed.), *International university reading course*. Nottingham: International University Society.

Beckenham, M. (1969). *Opening speech*. Paper presented at the Australian and New Zealand Association of Teachers of the Visually Handicapped Conference, Sydney.

Blatch, P. (1989). *The decentralisation of educational programs for visually handicapped students in Queensland*. Unpublished master's thesis, University of Queensland.

Blatch, P., Nagel, G., & Cruickshank, L. (1998). Current practices and future directions. In P. Kelley, & G. Gale (Eds.), *Towards excellence: Effective education for students with vision impairments*. North Rocks, NSW: North Rocks Press, pp. 17-18.

Cleverley, J. F. (1971). *The first generation*. Sydney: Sydney University Press.

Crawford, R. M. (1979). *Australia*. Sydney: Hutchinson of Australia.

Davidson, T. M. (1966). *A historical study of an aspect of Victorian education: Education of the visually handicapped, 1867-1950*. Melbourne: University of Melbourne unpublished paper.

Deaf and Dumb Institution of New South Wales. (1870). *First anniversary to ninth anniversary annual reports*. Sydney: Joseph Cook and Co.

Hunt, C. C. (1984). *Masonic concordance of the Holy Bible*. Bloomington, IL: The Masonic Book Club.

Kauffman, J. (1980). Historical trends and contemporary issues in special education in the United States. In J. Kauffman, & D. Hallahan (Eds), *Handbook of Special Education*. New York: Prentice-Hall, pp. 3-23.

Kelley, P., & Gale, G. M. (Eds). (1998). *Towards excellence: Effective education for students with vision impairments.* North Rocks, NSW: North Rocks Press.

Kelley, P., Gale, G. M., & Cruickshank, L. (1998). Historical development in the education of students with vision impairments. In P. Kelley, & G. Gale (Eds), *Towards excellence: Effective education for students with vision impairments.* North Rocks, NSW: North Rocks Press.

Law, A. (1922). *How the Church came to us in Australia.* Melbourne: Imperial Press.

McCaskie, J. (1973). *Royal Victorian Institute for the Blind, 1866-1973.* Unpublished historical study for the Royal Victorian Institute for the Blind.

Moores, D. F. (1996). *Educating the deaf: Psychology, principles, and practices.* Palo Alto, CA: Houghton Mifflin Company.

Murphy, I. F. (1965). *The education of the blind in South Australia.* Unpublished bachelor's thesis. University of Adelaide.

New South Wales Department of Education. (1974). *New South Wales Department of Education.* Sydney, NSW: Department of Education.

New South Wales Department of School Education. (1997). *Vision impairment: A reference for schools, Section 1.* Sydney: Author.

Nuske, A. (Ed.). (1992). *The years between: An oral history of he Royal Victorian Institute for the Blind, 1866 to 1991.* Melbourne: Royal Victorian Institute for the Blind.

Plowman, J. (1985). *We grew up together.* North Rocks, NSW: North Rocks Press.

Potts, A. (1999). Public and private schooling in Australia. *Phi Delta Kappan, November*, pp. 242-245.

Pritchard, C. (1997). *The development of a religious ethos in non-Catholic independent secondary schools, 1858-1959.* Nedlands, WA: Unpublished MEd thesis, University of Western Australia.

Rich, P. J. (1991). Perth's "The Cloisters" as an icon of educational elitism: Romancing the stone. *Education Research and Perspectives*, 18(1), 1-6.

Scholl, G. (1986). *Foundations of education for blind and visually handicapped youth.* New York: American Foundation for the Blind.

Steer, M. (2000). Moon code: A valuable supplement to your communications arsenal. *Deaf-Blind Perspectives*, Spring, 8-10.

Trewin, D. (2002). 2002 *Australian year book.* Canberra: Australian Bureau of Statistics.

Turney, C. (Ed.). (1975). *Sources in the history of Australian education, 1788-1870.* Sydney: Angus and Robertson.

Watkins, K. W. (1987). *Towards systematic education of the blind in Australia.* Unpublished doctoral dissertation, Macquarie University, Sydney.

Western Australian Council for Special Education. (1978). *Education of visually handicapped children in Western Australia.* Perth: Author.

Wilson, B. (1957). The first bishop: Mathew Hale. In F. Alexander (Ed.), *Four bishops and their See. Perth, Western Australia 1857-1957.* Nedlands, WA: University of Western Australia Press.

Recognizing All Members:
The Place of People with Disabilities
in the Uniting Church in Australia

Ann Wansbrough, BA, BSc, BD (Hons.), PhD, DipEd
Nicola Cooper, BAppScOT, MPH

SUMMARY. In this article, we present a case study related to the New South Wales (NSW) Synod of the Uniting Church in Australia (UCA). We look at the gap between the official theology of the Church and its

---

Reverend Dr. Ann Wansbrough is a theologian and Principal Policy Analyst for UnitingCare NSW.ACT, an agency of the Uniting Church in Australia. She was recently responsible for the NSW Synod's substantial statement, Directions for Health Policy. She has had a personal interest in disability issues since she became an amputee while at theological college in 1974. She is Co-Chair of the Social Justice Network of the National Council of Churches in Australia. Contact: Rev. Dr. Ann Wansbrough, P.O. Box A 2178, Sydney South, NSW, 1235, Australia (E-mail: annw@nsw.uca.org.au).

Nicola Cooper is a member of the Uniting Church. She has a Bachelor of Applied Science in Occupational Therapy and is currently undertaking a Master of Public Health degree at the University of Sydney. In 2001 she commenced the pilot project on disability access in the Uniting Church NSW Synod, and wrote the Action Plan for the congregations within the NSW Synod. She was an advisor on the 2002 Uniting Church Synod Arrangements Committee, and continues to be on this committee.

Address correspondence to: Ms. Nicola Cooper, 4/14 Crows Nest Road, Waverton, NSW 2060, Australia (E-mail: t4224t@bigpond.com).

[Haworth co-indexing entry note]: "Recognizing All Members: The Place of People with Disabilities in the Uniting Church in Australia." Wansbrough, Ann, and Nicola Cooper. Co-published simultaneously in *Journal of Religion, Disability & Health* (The Haworth Pastoral Press, an imprint of The Haworth Press, Inc.) Vol. 8, No. 1/2, 2004, pp. 145-165; and: *Voices in Disability and Spirituality from the Land Down Under: Outback to Outfront* (ed: Christopher Newell, and Andy Calder) The Haworth Pastoral Press, an imprint of The Haworth Press, Inc., 2004, pp. 145-165. Single or multiple copies of this article are available for a fee from The Haworth Document Delivery Service [1-800-HAWORTH, 9:00 a.m. - 5:00 p.m. (EST). E-mail address: docdelivery@haworthpress.com].

http://www.haworthpress.com/web/JRDH
Digital Object Identifier: 10.1300/J095v8n01_12

145

policy and practice, compare this to the Church's approach to other groups who have experienced barriers to Church participation, and outline a project which is attempting to move the Church forward to a more appropriate praxis. *[Article copies available for a fee from The Haworth Document Delivery Service: 1-800-HAWORTH. E-mail address: <docdelivery@ haworthpress.com> Website: <http://www.HaworthPress.com> © 2004 by The Haworth Press, Inc. All rights reserved.]*

KEYWORDS. Uniting Church, disability, policy, practice

INTRODUCTION

This case study is based on a view that people with disabilities are not 'differently abled' but are part of a wide diversity of Uniting Church members. The barriers that they face in the Church stem from a lack of awareness of how to deal with practical problems, rather than from an inherent difference created by their disability.

A particular methodology also underlies the case study, which is about praxis, the way we operate and the ideas that support that. If the Church is to move from unjust to just praxis, then we need to pay attention to specific experiences of injustice, analyze and question the ideas that support the injustice, recover those parts of the Christian tradition that will help us understand the demands of justice on these specific issues, determine the principles that justice requires as the basis for future action, and take action to bring about change (Wansbrough, 2000). This is not a simple or linear process; rather there is interaction between these tasks. The point is that change does not come from sweeping generalizations and grand abstractions, but from dealing with reality and finding ideas that have value in bringing about change in particular contexts.

While we refer to specific Uniting Church documents, we believe that neither the issues of praxis nor the theology of the UCA documents are unique to the UCA. The case study is offered as a way of assisting people in all Churches sharpen the way they deal with these issues.

FUNDAMENTALS OF OUR FAITH

'Differently Abled,' or Part of a Wide 'Diversity'?

In 1995, the late Elizabeth Hastings, then commissioner for disability with Australia's Human Rights and Equal Opportunity Commission, launched the disability policy of the NSW Synod of the Uniting Church in Australia. She questioned the title of the document, "Include me in." Her concern was that it implied that people with disabilities are a separate group, not yet part of the Church. She was an Anglican who had a disability, addressing a Uniting Church synod that included some people with disabilities. The title clearly gave a false impression. The situation of those who face barriers to full participation because of disabilities is not helped by giving the impression that we disabled are outside, rather than inside, the Church. Expressions like 'include me in' also sound like a plea to those in power; as if the Church has the right to decide who belongs and who does not. Instead, language and policy should reflect that people with disabilities belong, enhance respect, and help people see the wrongness of the barriers and harms that they encounter in the life of the Church.

This example illustrates why the question of how to talk about people with disabilities theologically is of fundamental importance. Inadequate and inappropriate concepts can be offensive and encourage ideas that support discrimination and injustice. Appropriate theology can help the Church see situations and issues clearly, and can assist in ending discrimination and harm.

An examination of the synod policy shows that it is not only the title that is problematic. There are generalizations such as "people with disabilities constitute a community that makes space for God" and "people with disabilities teach others that there is more to ministry than clinical understanding." These comments are not only unrealistic; they also sanctify disability. They give people with disabilities characteristics and responsibilities based on their disability, instead of recognizing the characteristics they share with other human beings and with other Christians. The same impression is given in the section on inclusive ministry in the congregation. The basic assumption seems to be that people with disabilities and people who are not 'disabled' are different and complementary.

This approach to the question of disability is not unique, of course, to this policy document. It seems to be the view of Moltmann, for example, when he argues that the non-handicapped and the handicapped need one another and that there is need for change "on both sides" (Moltmann, 1983, p. 150). The same view seems to underlie the term 'differently abled' which is used by the World Council of Churches and elsewhere.

The problem with a theology of 'difference,' or complementarity, is that it conveys the impression that disability changes the nature of one's humanity. Disability becomes the basis of one's humanity and one's participation in the Church. This undermines some of the central theology of the Christian faith.

Church membership is not primarily about human action, but about God's action–through Christ, through baptism, through the work of the Holy Spirit. The issue of participation is not about letting disabled people in, but about acknowledging the reality of God's Church, in which we disabled are present, and removing the practical barriers that stand in the way of our full participation.

Ministers with a Diversity of Gifts

This attempt to create a special theology is puzzling in a Uniting Church document. A more appropriate approach would have been to start with the Basis of Union, the document that formed the basis on which Methodist, Presbyterian, and Congregationalist Churches became the Uniting Church in Australia in 1977.

The Basis of Union recognizes that it is God who calls people, both women and men, to Ministry of the Word, to the ministries of elder and lay preacher, and to the roles required for the government of the Church. It is God, through the Holy Spirit, who gives people the appropriate gifts for the ministry to which they are called. It is not the role of the Church to categorize people and determine what part they can play. It is the role of the Church to listen to God, to recognize those to whom God has given the particular gifts of the Spirit that are required for particular roles and tasks, and to "*order its life*" in an appropriate way so that it uses the gifts of ministry that God gives to people (par. 13).

Each council of the Church (congregation, presbytery, synod, and assembly) has the responsibility "to wait upon God's Word and to obey God's will in the matters allocated to its oversight" (par. 15). This recognition of the local congregation as a council of the Church is crucial to Uniting Church understanding of participation and ministry. Every member of the Church has one or more God-given gifts of ministry. The Church needs to both recognize the gifts and provide ways in which the person can exercise the appropriate ministry that utilizes those gifts. No one can be left out. No one is without a ministry. No one has a 'special ministry' because of disability. Everyone has a ministry, a special ministry, by virtue of their God-given gifts and the responsibilities that go with the gift. So, in the Uniting Church, we talk about specified ministries (for which professional training is required and certain status is granted through ordination and induction, or commissioning) and lay ministry (for which the Church offers less formal training and different forms of recognition). It is all ministry, it is all important, and it often overlaps.

Fellowship of Reconciliation

This theology of ministry is consistent throughout the Basis of Union. It is shaped by Christology. Jesus is "a representative beginning of a new order of righteousness and love" (par. 3). The Church is a fellowship of reconciliation, "a body within which the diverse gifts of its members are used for the building up of the whole, an instrument through which Christ may work and bear witness to himself" (par. 3). All ministry and the whole life of the Church depends on Jesus Christ, "who gives life to the dead and brings into being what otherwise could not exist" (par. 4).

The Basis of Union describes Baptism as Christ's act, the way Christ incorporates people into his own baptism, the benefits of his saving work in life, death, and resurrection, and the gift of the Holy Spirit. "Baptism into Christ's body initiates people into Christ's life and mission in the world" (par. 7). Through the Holy Communion or Eucharist, people "grow together into Christ, are strengthened for their participation in the mission of God in the world, and rejoice in the foretaste of the Kingdom which Christ will bring to consummation" (par. 8).

This understanding of salvation, membership, and mission renders a theology of the 'differently abled' unnecessary and counter-productive. Ministry belongs to the whole people of God. For the Uniting Church, being the Church means ordering our life together so that all may participate, so that we value all as fellow Christians. We are to value the gifts God has given each and every member and ensure that they are used in an appropriate ministry. If we as a Church are to be faithful to the Basis of Union, we cannot define people's ministry on the basis of characteristics such as age, sex, or disability and we cannot allow barriers to remain that prevent anyone from using their gifts in an appropriate ministry. We people with disabilities belong in the Church, and participate in its life, on the same grounds, for the same purposes, and with the same range of gifts of the Spirit as anyone else.

EVALUATING PRAXIS

UCA Models in Other Areas of Diversity

The UCA commitment to recognizing God's diverse gifts and the ministries of all members is reflected in regulations, policy, and practice. As the Basis of Union and the Constitution and Regulations were developed, some attention was paid to some groups who had faced barriers in the Churches proposing union–non-clergy, women, and people of youthful age.

The UCA regulations require that the national assembly, synods, and presbyteries have at least as many non-ordained as ordained members. Both women and men may be ordained. There is no Church structure by which ordained clergy alone can control ("guide," "lead," or "serve") the Church or its agencies and activities. Both ordained and non-ordained men and women have occupied leadership roles such as president, moderator, synod secretary, executive directors of official Church agencies, and chairperson and secretary of presbytery. The only role that is usually reserved for ordained ministers is the celebration of the Eucharist, but a presbytery can allocate this role to a layperson if the person has the appropriate gifts and training and the presbytery believes that circumstances warrant them exercising this role. The Basis of Union provided for at least one third of various councils and committees to be women for the first years of its life. That provision was later extended. It also provided for the participation of people of youthful age.

Later decisions have also been aimed at encouraging and enabling participation of all. In 1985 the assembly adopted the policy that children, as baptized members of the Church, should receive the Eucharist. In more recent times, the Church has developed programs to enable children to participate in synod and assembly as voting members. The children's education policy recognizes that children are Church members and this should shape their education. The national Assembly has adopted policies seeking to give appropriate power over their own congregations and ministers to Indigenous members of the Church (by establishing the Uniting Aboriginal and Islander Christian Congress in 1985, and by other means). The 1985 statement, *The Uniting Church is a Multicultural Church*, was intended to move the Church towards ensuring participation of migrant-ethnic groups in the Church, especially those of non-English speaking backgrounds. The Church has also adopted a consensus process for decision-making (*A Manual for Meetings, 1994*). Its aim is to ensure that views are shared in the course of large meetings such as synod and assembly and that people have the chance to contribute on the basis of their gifts and insights rather than status. Programs such as covenanting and cross-cultural awareness workshops help people understand how their personal behavior needs to change to allow others to participate.

The Church has thus sought to order its life to allow identified groups of people who have previously been disadvantaged to enter fully into the life of the Church and participate in its power structures. None of the structures or mechanisms is perfect, but they do represent significant progress and changed norms. Struggles are not at the level of arguing theologically that these groups should participate and have the right to participate (include me in); the struggle is to improve Church practice.

UCA and People with Disabilities

There are two groups for whom the UCA has failed to take seriously the theology of membership and ministry in the Basis of Union. These are people with disabilities and people who are homosexual. In both cases, the problem is the wrong focus on a theology of difference. In both cases, it appears to want to make rules that override the clear evidence that God gives gifts of ministry to all Christians; it is not on the basis of rules determined by the Church on the basis of categories. Here we will consider only people with disabilities.

Since 1980, the NSW Synod of the Uniting Church has had policy resolutions committing it to make churches and other buildings accessible. There are some examples of new and refurbished buildings providing for the needs of people with disabilities. Yet, in recent years, churches have been built that provide access for people in wheelchairs into the building but not into the sanctuary and pulpit of the church, nor onto the stage in the hall. This suggests a view that people with disabilities can participate in the sense of attend, but not lead. The synod's building advisory committee has in the past seemed more concerned with cost than in finding practicable solutions. Many Church buildings continue to be so badly sign-posted that it is difficult to find the wheelchair entrance or toilet. When UnitingCare NSW.ACT employed a person in a wheelchair as a disability officer, some 20 years after Church union, she could access the building to work, but had to go to the building next door to use the toilet.

Synod and assembly meetings have been held in buildings with limited accessibility either to the auditorium, the stage, the small group meeting rooms, the toilets, the catering facilities, or all of these. In 1995, Elizabeth Hastings had to launch the NSW Synod disability policy from the floor of the auditorium because there was no way to get her wheelchair onto the stage. Some people with disabilities have found that they were unable to attend the meetings of national committees to which they were appointed, because they were held at inaccessible venues. In 2002, the NSW Synod held its meeting at the Canterbury Race Course, an accessible venue, and there was an advisor on access issues in the Synod Arrangements Committee, 2002.

At the beginning of the 1990's, the NSW synod was asked to set up a task group to look at the circumstances under which a person with a disability might be allowed to be a candidate for the ordained ministry. This was clearly discriminatory, and the synod instead passed a resolution to look at the obstacles which ministers with disabilities face, and how the obstacles might be removed. Whereas synod would require that a task group about women or Indigenous people included a number of those people, in this case the task group included only one minister with a disability. The task group did not consult with each of the ministers with disabilities. The report was phrased in terms of making concessions to ministers with disabilities, rather than in accordance with the theology of the Basis of Union.

Both the process and the report involved discrimination, and perpetrated the stereotype of people with disabilities as different, dependent, and burdensome. This is disturbing. Ordained ministers have gone through a rigorous process of selection, education, and assessment as to their readiness for ministry. The UCA invests considerable money and time in training them. Many have two or more degrees. It is in its own interests to remove any barriers that ordained ministers with disabilities encounter in their ministry. It is both theologically wrong and a waste of resources to fail to do so. If the Church cannot get past stereotypes and embrace the theology of the basis of union regarding ordained ministers, then the situation is likely to be even more difficult for non-ordained people with disabilities.

The Community, Disability, and Ageing Program, University of Sydney, measured Uniting Church attitudes towards disability at a disability awareness workshop in 1996. The score on the 'Interaction with Disabled Persons Scale' showed that the Uniting Church participants' perceived level of discomfort when interacting was lower than the general population (Cahill, 1996, p. 7). "Community attitudes towards people with disabilities are widely regarded as being negative. [Attitudes interfere] with quality of life and acceptance . . . as valued members of the community" (Gething, 1994, p. 23). Negative attitudes towards people with disabilities are likely to hinder full participation in society. Despite the level of acceptance being higher in the Uniting Church than in the community, inclusion of people with disabilities remains a pressing issue, as our other examples show.

In 1998, the Board for Social Responsibility (now UnitingCare NSW.ACT) and the Board of Education of the NSW Synod issued the *Disability Education and Services Policy*. This is about discrimination in society as well as the Church. It focuses on the Church's solidarity with people who suffer injustice, in the Church's service provision and advocacy. It requires that all Church-run disability services include people with disabilities in their management. However, its section on "the faith context" still focuses on difference and talks about the need for inclusion.

In 1998 the Synod employed two suitably qualified people with disabilities as Disability Education and Service Officers. Their work demonstrated a need to address the problem of access into congregations. In 2001, the Church advertised for an Access Officer to oversee the access project outlined later in this article. A person who mobilizes in a wheelchair was unsuccessful, partly because he would not be able to access all the churches in the pilot project.

Clearly, in relation to people with disabilities, there is room for improvement in the Church's praxis. For the UCA, what is at stake is its adherence to the Basis of Union, something that all those in specified ministry have undertaken in their ordination vows. The development of the Action Plan reported in the next section is clearly essential if the Church is to improve its praxis.

IMPROVING PRAXIS–THE ACTION PLAN

The development of the action plan in NSW has been quite different from the approach adopted by the Victorian Synod, which also has an action plan.

The Legal Context

In Australia, the human rights of people with disabilities are enforced by the *Disability Discrimination Act 1992* (DDA), which is administered by the Human Rights and Equal Opportunity Commission (HREOC). One of HREOC's responsibilities is to advise organizations on the development of Action Plans and to register these plans. Plans are voluntary, but registering and implementing plans is a way of demonstrating compliance with the act.

In defining disability in the DDA, Australia rejected the restrictive "major life activity" requirement found in USA and UK legislation. Instead, it adopted a generally more pragmatic approach (Innis, 2000).

The categories of disability within the DDA include total or partial loss of the person's bodily or mental function; total or partial loss of part of the body; the presence in the body of organisms capable of causing disease or mental illness; malfunction, malformation, or disfigurement of part of a person's body; a disorder or malfunctioning that results in differences in learning; and a disorder, illness, or disease that affects a person's thought process, perceptions of reality, emotions or judgement, and results in disturbed behavior. A person's disabilities are covered by the Act if they presently exist, if they have previously existed, if they may exist in the future or if they are imputed to the person.

The DDA proposes action plans as a mechanism for eliminating discrimination and promoting equality within organizations. They generally focus on preventing discrimination and addressing currently known barriers to discrimination; sometimes ignoring the value of complaints mechanisms in bringing about change (Innes, 2000).

Developing action plans is consistent with the theology of the Uniting Church and can usefully shape the approach taken by the Church. The NSW Synod has created an Action Plan. In October 2001, an access officer, who was an occupational therapist, was employed to initiate an access pilot project by working with congregations to develop local action plans. This plan recommends that the Synod ensure that:

- congregations understand that people with disabilities have a right (ethically and legally) to be included in worship, activities, and decision-making

- complaints about equity and access are considered with sensitivity and are acted upon when upheld
- when any changes occur, people with disabilities must have the opportunity to be involved in the consultation process
- when new facilities are under consideration, relevant design standards will be met

The vision for the project is that Uniting Church buildings, worship, and activities will be welcoming and accessible to all people and will enable their participation, and that the Church's understanding of gifts and ministry, as outlined in the Basis of Union, will be achieved. Removing barriers enables participation and service, thereby moving closer to acknowledging that the one spirit has endowed the members of Christ's Church with a diversity of gifts and that there is no gift without its corresponding service.

Aims

The project aimed to:

- make a workable action plan to be followed by congregations
- provide education regarding disability issues
- provide an estimation of costs involved, and create an appropriate loans system

The Action Plan is due to be endorsed at the March 2003 Council of Synod, after which it will be submitted to the Human Rights and Equal Opportunity Commission.

The Congregations

The study included members of eight congregations. Its emphasis was on people who are elderly and people with disabilities. The National Church Life Survey of 2001 showed that in the Uniting Church, the percentage of people over sixty years of age is 56%. Elderly people were included within the study, because their changing health needs create changing needs for access.

The congregations were chosen on the basis of their building type, multi-ethnic mix, and activities of the congregation. It is a purposive sample. Two churches have Tongan congregations, and one, a Korean congregation. Congregation activities included meals programs, literacy programs, after-school care, adult groups, and counseling.

Developing the Plan

Pilot project activities and their advantages are enumerated below:

1. Focus groups allowed in-depth discussion of issues with a small group of participants.
2. An access audit of the architectural features of the building provided practical solutions and costs.
3. A questionnaire regarding access covered more topics and allowed anonymous views to be expressed by a wider population.
4. Education packages regarding issues of disability were made to foster inclusion.
5. An action plan was created and provides a practical means of addressing identified barriers to access.

Focus Groups

Access Australia, a consultancy firm that specializes in access, ran the focus groups and performed the building audits. The consultants were an occupational therapist and an architect. Focus groups aimed to:

- inform the participants of the provisions of the DDA
- identify the current social, attitudinal, and physical access barriers to inclusion of people with disabilities within the congregation
- seek the preferences of people with disabilities for overcoming (identified) barriers

In practice, focus groups concentrated on the provisions of the DDA, plus physical and sensory access issues. Social, attitudinal, and cognitive issues were not covered in detail. Five to thirteen members participated; in the larger groups not all members contributed to the discussion. All ethnic-migrant congregations were offered translators; only the Korean congregation accepted.

Access Audits

Churches, halls, kitchens, toilet facilities, and other areas were audited. The benchmarking standards used were:

- Australian Standards AS 1428 Part 1: Design for access and mobility: General requirements for access–New building work

- Australian Standards AS 1428 Part 2: Design for access and mobility: Enhanced and additional requirements–Buildings and facilities
- Australian Standard AS 2890 Part 1: Parking facilities
- The Building Code of Australia (BCA)
- Austroads, Part 13: Traffic engineering practice, Pedestrians
- Advisory Notes on Access to Premises, June 1997, Human Rights and Equal Opportunity Commission

Audit reports prioritized solutions with respect to safety, equity, and dignity, and the likelihood of an event occurring.

Education Packages

Education packages, based on requested information and identified problems, were compiled. It is intended that they will increase congregations' knowledge and, therefore, ability to include people with disabilities.

Action Plan

The action plan was created from the above-mentioned research. It outlines problems with access, solutions, time frames for implementing solutions, and monitoring processes, and asks congregations to identify relevant committees responsible for implementing and monitoring solutions. It includes a complaints mechanism that will aid in fostering change. The resources provided with the action plan provide information related to a range of physical and mental disabilities.

Questionnaire

A questionnaire was developed by the Access Officer with the assistance of Professor Susan Quine, the Associate Professor of Community Medicine at the University of Sydney. The questionnaire was a pre-test tool. Pilot congregations have individualized post-test questionnaires to measure the effectiveness of interventions and education. The questionnaire consisted of mutually exclusive, nominal questions; Likert scales; open ended and closed questions. It addresses the following:

- The age of the respondent
- Whether or not the respondent has a disability that is physical, mental, or both
- Attitude towards congregation members with physical and mental disabilities

- Whether or not members feel included and valued within the congregation
- Process of the worship service
- Can the individuals hear, see, and use the worship materials
- Whether or not the seating arrangements foster inclusion
- If people are given time to express themselves and if their language needs are met
- Help that is available and help that is needed for carers
- Aspects of disability about which respondents would like to have more information

Questionnaire Results

Response Rate

Out of 365 questionnaires that were sent out, there were 195 responses: a response rate of 53%.

Characteristics of Respondents

- Elderly people (over 65 years of age): 122 respondents (62%)
- People with disabilities: 47 respondents (24%)
- People with physical disabilities: 41 respondents (21%)
- People with mental disabilities: 5 respondents (3%)
- People with mental and physical disabilities: 2 respondents (1%)
- Elderly people with disabilities: 40 respondents 20%)

These percentages can be compared with the estimated disability rate in the general population of 19% (Australian Bureau of Statistics, 2000) and 1.5% with mental health problems at any one time (Human Rights and Equal Opportunity Commission, 1992). The responses from all the congregations are tabulated below. Not all people responded to all the questions; therefore, the numbers do not add up to 195.

Do People in the Uniting Church Value People with a Disability?

Table 1 shows that 97% of those who answered the question said they valued people with physical disability, and 84% of those who answered the question said they valued people with mental disability. This is a very positive result. It was also a surprising result, given the number of access problems that exist in these congregations and in the wider Uniting Church. The congregations have begun imple-

TABLE 1. I Value People with a

	Strongly Disagree	Disagree	Undecided	Strongly Agree	Agree
Physical disability			4	90	96
Mental disability		1	30	92	72

menting the action plan; even more, it has been adopted by synod (Cooper, 2003). This suggests that their answers to this question were sincere.

More people were undecided about whether they value people with a mental disability than were undecided about valuing people with a physical disability (15% compared to 2%). There are two possible explanations. The first is that the result is an artifact of the study: people were not clear as to what was meant by mental disability (does it mean, for example, mental illness? or intellectual development disability? or dementia?), and their answers reflected that uncertainty rather than an uncertainty about attitudes. Alternatively, this 'undecidedness' may reveal that some people are still coming to terms with the concept of mental disability. Congregation members may feel more comfortable with physical disability than mental disability; they may know more people with physical disability and therefore have a greater understanding and comfort level about physical disability. Discomfort with mental illness creates barriers for inclusion. It reduces the chance of relationships forming, whereby each person has a chance to value and be valued, and where gifts can be given and received.

Some of the comments made at other points in this project suggest that, for some people at least, the second explanation may be correct. For example, some people expressed ambivalence about people with mental illness who from time to time exhibited disruptive behavior during worship or other activities. It may be that the answer "undecided" indicates that members of the Church are not willing to describe their attitude as not valuing people, but wanted to indicate that they face some difficulties in dealing with some people with mental disability. Resources in the action plan should assist congregations in overcoming these perceived difficulties.

Do People in the Uniting Church Who Are Elderly or Have a Disability Feel Valued by Their Congregation?

Table 2 shows that of those who responded to the question, 89% of all respondents felt valued by the congregation, compared to 95% of those who were elderly, 100% of those with a disability, and 91% of those who were both elderly and had a disability. Ten percent of all respondents were undecided as to whether they felt valued, compared to 5% of those who were elderly, none

TABLE 2. I Feel Valued by the Congregation

	Strongly Disagree	Disagree	Undecided	Agree	Strongly Agree
All responses		1	19	81	89
People who are elderly			2	15	26
People with a disability				1	10
People who are elderly and have a disability		1	3	17	13

of those with a disability, and 3% of those who were elderly and had a disability. The one person (0.5% of all respondents) who disagreed with the statement of being valued was both elderly and had a disability (3% of this category).

These results are very positive. They should not, however, be taken to mean that people who are elderly or have disabilities do not struggle to participate in the life of the congregation or that there is no need to improve accessibility and attitudes. The project as a whole revealed serious deficits in accessibility and practice.

Other parts of the project involved discussing with congregations how they might better value people with disabilities. Congregations themselves recognized that they needed to do better. The solutions offered by the congregations to help people with disabilities feel more valued included not focusing on their disability, and keeping in touch. One congregation member replied: "have a variety of forms of activities at worship so all can take part [and] involve [people with disabilities] to the limits of their abilities, [as] each of us have some gifts to offer." This is also a positive expression of the theology in the Basis of Union.

Do People Who Are Elderly and People Who Have a Disability Feel Included in Their Congregation?

Table 3 shows that of those who responded to the question, 98% of all respondents felt included in the congregation, compared to 100% of those who were elderly, 81% of those with a disability, and 97% of those who were elderly and had a disability. The three people who disagreed with the statement of inclusion constituted 2% of the total sample. Two of them had a disability (18% of the respondents with a disability), and one was elderly and had a disability (3% of the respondents in that category).

TABLE 3. I Feel Included in the Congregation

	Strongly Disagree	Disagree	Undecided	Strongly Agree	Agree
All responses	1	2	1	69	107
People who are elderly				12	31
People with a disability	1	1		3	6
People who are elderly and have a disability		1		15	18

Again, these results, while positive, cannot be taken to show that accessibility does not affect people's relationship to the Church, or that the Church is fully implementing its theology. Two respondents reported about physical access:

> I am an amputee and cannot get back to my church without [accessible] toilet facilities or a ramp.

> Provision of a reasonable means of access to church services and facilities [is necessary]. I have been with this congregation for over sixty years . . . [and] am very disappointed that because of disability (use of a wheelchair), I can no longer attend.

It is apparent that lack of access is preventing these congregation members from attending church, enjoying their rights, and fulfilling their responsibilities as members of the congregation. Where once, their faith and gifts defined their role in the Church, now their disability does. It must be assumed that many other people with similar disabilities are also unable to access the church.

In answer to an open-ended question to members of the congregations about inclusion, there were many suggestions. These ranged from communication issues to physical access. Suggestions to improve the former were to "be kept more up to date" and to have a "more face-to-face approach." This is a matter of greater effort rather than cost.

Other people may attend church but still face barriers to participation; for example, difficulty reading the overhead screen and poor lighting, not knowing that a hearing loop is available, or seating arrangements that isolate them.

A More Just Form of Participation

The results in Tables 2 and 3 are highly positive. People feel valued and included; even most of those who are elderly and/or have a disability. How are we to interpret this, given that we know, and the congregations acknowledge, that access needs to be improved?

Many elderly people bring with them a lifetime of Church experience and a faith that has been nurtured over many years. Their answers to these questions are best taken as showing that their sense of value and inclusion are based on much more than their current experience of accessibility. It may be partly based on their experience when they were younger or before they acquired a disability. But this finding also goes to the heart of the issue raised by Elizabeth Hastings, referred to at the beginning of this article. The Church does include people with disability. The problem has never been as simple as saying that lack of adequate access means people with disabilities are not valued or are unable to be part of the Church. The problem has been that the Church relies on people with disabilities making the effort to overcome the barriers. That is what the access project is intended to change–now the Church will make that effort. In many aspects of the Church's life, it is not about moving from exclusion to inclusion, but about moving from unjust conditions for participation to just conditions for participation. Unjust barriers are to be removed. The Church will no longer expect people with disabilities to be so forgiving of its failures and insensitivity.

The Action Plans

A local action plan was provided to each congregation that participated in the pilot study, and these are already being implemented. The information from the various processes was used to formulate a synod-wide action plan for congregations. It covers issues, goals, strategies, time frame, suggested responsible body, and ways of monitoring implementation. It includes an accessibility action plan, an access checklist, a list of resources, information on funding, information on international symbols, and resources relating to communication and hearing, communication and vision, mobility and wheelchairs, mobility and vision, epilepsy, dementia, Parkinson's Disease, stroke, head injury, intellectual disability, multiple sclerosis, depression, and schizophrenia. It is thus designed to be a comprehensive plan.

The action plan has acknowledged that heritage listed churches need special consideration; however, this does not exempt them from taking steps to improve access. Other issues covered in the action plan are: creating a formalized complaints mechanism; providing an accessible path of travel to the church and hall from accessible car park facilities; installing, maintaining, and advertising the presence of hearing augmentation systems; printing all overheads and handouts using large print guidelines; provision of integrated seating; and information about the accessible facilities of each church, to welcome visitors more effectively.

The action plan has not yet been lodged with HREOC. Despite this, the pilot congregations have taken steps to rectify problems identified for their building or worship processes. Such steps include increasing the print and font size of the worship sheets and handouts; linking the lapel microphone to the hearing loop system; provision of chairs with arm rests, accessible car parks, integrated seating and demountable ramps; installation of rails on both sides of the stair entrances; and liaison with local councils regarding provision of footpaths and/or curb ramps on government owned land adjoining Church property.

When the action plan is lodged with HREOC, all Uniting Churches in the NSW Synod will be expected to follow the action plan to improve access. The actions already taken by the pilot congregations are a positive example for other congregations, and attest to the commitment of congregations to make their Church buildings and process more accessible and more inclusive to people with disabilities. They show that congregations want to keep faith with the people who face problems of access and participation but who have nevertheless said that they feel valued and included.

Financial Feasibility

Every pilot congregation raised funding concerns. One respondent stated that "congregations must be prepared to spend money on better access for people with disabilities, including wheelchair users."

Congregations with activities such as the meals programs have stated, "government regulations to enforce standards (for example, provision of heating trays) add to our budget constraints, as funding is only from the Church." Other congregations have found proposed modifications too costly. For example, quotes have reached $43,740 (AUS) for installation of mechanical lifts. Therefore, other options need consideration.

Where buildings are multi-level or have a close proximity to other buildings, creating permanent standard ramps is often not possible. In one such congregation a de-mountable ramp is used, and installed with prior notice. This prevents people who use wheelchairs entering church spontaneously.

Many churches are heritage buildings. One person stated that they "try hard to retain [the church's] heritage fabric, to honor the congregation and the city." Full access to heritage buildings may not be possible. It is important to:

> . . . evaluate accessibility options within a conservation context . . . Solutions should provide the greatest level of access without adverse effects

on the place's significance. Solutions should also minimize modifications, as this reduces their impact and, often, their cost. (Martin, 1999)

As a result of this project, the Board of Finance and Property has developed a loans system to help congregations finance the modifications required by the Action Plan.

Signs of Hope

During the project, positive progress in creating an accessible church for people with disabilities has been observed. This augurs well for inclusion of people with disabilities and creating access on a wider scale than the pilot congregations. Church members have become more aware that people with disabilities face issues when joining congregation activities and using Church buildings. Members of congregations have asked many questions and made many phone calls to inquire about how to deal with access issues that the congregations have identified for themselves. Congregations outside the project have also inquired about modifications to Church buildings and Church processes. The pilot congregations all affirmed that they wanted to include people with disabilities better, identified gaps in their knowledge about disability issues, and requested relevant information. All the congregations acted upon many problems identified on the initial visit to their church prior to the action plan being provided. Some congregations have discussed instituting pastoral care committees, to be more proactive about meeting the needs of all their members. The acceptance and action taken so far are positive indicators that other congregation members will seize the opportunity to make their activities inclusive, and buildings accessible to all.

CONCLUSION

There is no doubt that the Uniting Church needs an action plan to ensure accessibility for people with disabilities. At stake is the sincerity of its theology of membership and ministry, and its faithfulness in expressing the Gospel that it says it believes. This project has sought to provide an action plan that is clearly defined and capable of implementation. It will make a difference. There is now a loan system in place so congregations can afford to implement the plan.

While people with disabilities have good reason to criticize the inaccessibility of the Uniting Church in Australia, there is now reason for hope. Its theology of membership and ministry lays good foundations for people with disabilities to feel valued and included. The accessibility project shows that congregations can become committed to accessibility for everyone when provided with appropriate information, ideas, and means of funding.

The Basis of Union ends with an affirmation and a prayer:

> The Uniting Church affirms that it belongs to the people of God on the way to the promised end. The Uniting Church prays that, through the gift of the Spirit, God will constantly correct that which is erroneous in its life, will bring it into deeper unity with other Churches, and will use its worship, witness, and service to God's eternal glory through Jesus Christ the Lord. Amen.

To which people with disabilities will surely say Amen, and apply it not only to the Uniting Church but also to all Churches.

REFERENCES

Attorney General's Department. (1996). *Disability Discrimination Act 1992.* Australian Government Publishing Service, Canberra.

Australian Bureau of Statistics, 2001. *Disability, New South Wales: 2001.* Australian Bureau of Statistics, Canberra.

Cahill, L. (1996). Uniting Church Disability Awareness Workshop: Including people with disabilities. Community Disability Ageing Program. Sydney: University of Sydney.

Cooper N. (2003). *Access for people with disabilities: A guide to making your congregation more inclusive.* Sydney: UnitingCare NSW.ACT.

Eiseland, N. (1994). *The disabled God: Toward a liberatory theology.* Nashville: Abingdon Press.

Gething, L. (1994). The interaction with disabled persons scale. *Journal of Social Behavior and Personality,* vol. 9, no.5, pp. 23-42.

Human Rights and Equal Opportunity Commission. (1993). *Human rights and mental illness: Report of the National Inquiry into the Human Rights of People with Mental Illness, Volume 1.* Canberra: Australian Government Publishing Service.

Innes, G. (2000). *The role of public inquiries and exemption powers in eliminating disability discrimination.* Retrieved April 29, 2002, from: http://www.hreoc.gov.au/disability_rights/speeches/constructing.htm

Martin, E. (1999). *Improving access to heritage buildings: A practical guide to meeting the needs of people with disabilities.* Australian Heritage Commission. Retrieved February 5, 2002, from: http://www.ahc.gov.au/infores/publs/generalpubs/access/chapter2.html

Moltmann, J. (1983). The liberation and acceptance of the handicapped. *The power of the powerless: The word of liberation for today.* Toronto: Fitzhenry and Whiteside.

Newell, C., & Gillespie, F. (2001). Psychiatric disability and pastoral care: Towards a richer theology of disability. *Contact: The Interdisciplinary Journal of Pastoral*

Studies, no. 136. Edinburgh: Scottish Pastoral Association and Clinical Theology Association, pp. 5-13.

Uniting Church in Australia. (1992). Basis of Union. Retrieved from: http://nat.uca.org.au/basisofunion/Basis1992.htm

Uniting Church in Australia, Synod of Victoria. (2000). Disability Action Plan 2000-2003. Available from http://vic.unitingcare.org.au/

Wansbrough, A. (2000). *Speaking together: A methodology for the National Council of Churches contribution to public policy debate in Australia*. PhD thesis, Sydney University.

Index

equality of people with disabilities,
  69-73
Golden Rule, 71
high priest as Jewish hero, 71-73
justice, 77
law of inclusive social relations,
  71-79
Law of the Pursuer, 68-69
life as utmost value in, 66
and life not worth living concept,
  65
Life Saving Principle, 67-68
requirement to choose life, 66
spirituality and, 57-61,79-82
Stumbling Block Principle, 75-76
valuing people with disabilities,
  64-69
visiting the sick, 76-77

Make Today Count, 110
Marcel, Gabriel, 35
McGrath, Pam, 89-103
Memorial gardens, 111
Middleton, Laura, 111
Miraculous healing concept, 8-9
Mosely, Elizabeth, 115-124
Moses, 72

Newel, Christopher, 1-3,89-103
New South Wales, educational
  institutions for blind, 133-135
Non-verbal communication, 92-93

On Equilibrium (Saul), 29-30

Palette & Pen: A Healing Journey
  (Mosely), 115-124
Palliative care, 98
  Frederick's ataxia case study,
    89-103

Pastoral care, 5-19
  as advocacy, 15
  as community building, 16
  community spirit and, 105-114
  as companionship, 14-15
  as friendship, 17-18
Personal Advocacy Service, 125-128
*(A) Place to Belong: Building
  Welcoming Communities*
  (Anglicare report), 116
Poetry, 115-124
Protocols, community, 110

Queensland, educational institutions
  for blind, 138-139
Queensland Advocacy International,
  21-31
Queensland Cancer Fund study
  demographics, 91-92
  discussion, 98-103
  findings, 92-98
  research, 91

Receiving vs. giving, 125-128
Reid, Leonie, 125-128
Rejectivity, 41
Religiosity, vs. spirituality, 93-94

Shakenness, 41
South Australia, educational
  institutions for blind, 137-138
Spirituality
  antipodean perspective, 1-3
  Australian Jewry and, 79-82. *See
    also* Judaism
  Frederick's ataxia case study,
    89-103
  vs. religiosity, 93-94
Spirituality Revolution, The (Tacey),
  1-2

BOOK ORDER FORM!

Order a copy of this book with this form or online at:
http://www.haworthpress.com/store/product.asp?sku=5339

Voices in Disability and Spirituality
from the Land Down Under
Outback to Outfront

___ in softbound at $19.95 (ISBN: 0-7890-2608-2)
___ in hardbound at $39.95 (ISBN: 0-7890-2607-4)

COST OF BOOKS _____

POSTAGE & HANDLING _____
US: $4.00 for first book & $1.50
for each additional book.
Outside US: $5.00 for first book
& $2.00 for each additional book.

SUBTOTAL _____

In Canada: add 7% GST._____

STATE TAX _____
CA, IL, IN, MN, NY, OH & SD residents
please add appropriate local sales tax.

FINAL TOTAL _____

If paying in Canadian funds, convert
using the current exchange rate,
UNESCO coupons welcome.

❏ BILL ME LATER:
Bill-me option is good on US/Canada/
Mexico orders only; not good to jobbers,
wholesalers, or subscription agencies.

❏ Signature _____

❏ Payment Enclosed: $ _____

❏ PLEASE CHARGE TO MY CREDIT CARD:
❏ Visa ❏ MasterCard ❏ AmEx ❏ Discover
❏ Diner's Club ❏ Eurocard ❏ JCB

Account #_____

Exp Date _____

Signature _____
(Prices in US dollars and subject to change without notice.)

PLEASE PRINT ALL INFORMATION OR ATTACH YOUR BUSINESS CARD
Name
Address
City   State/Province   Zip/Postal Code
Country
Tel   Fax
E-Mail

May we use your e-mail address for confirmations and other types of information? ❏ Yes ❏ No We appreciate receiving
your e-mail address. Haworth would like to e-mail special discount offers to you, as a preferred customer.
We will never share, rent, or exchange your e-mail address. We regard such actions as an invasion of your privacy.

Order From Your **Local Bookstore** or Directly From
The Haworth Press, Inc. 10 Alice Street, Binghamton, New York 13904-1580 • USA
Call Our toll-free number (1-800-429-6784) / Outside US/Canada: (607) 722-5857
Fax: 1-800-895-0582 / Outside US/Canada: (607) 771-0012
E-mail your order to us: orders@haworthpress.com

For orders outside US and Canada, you may wish to order through your local
sales representative, distributor, or bookseller.
For information, see http://haworthpress.com/distributors

(Discounts are available for individual orders in US and Canada only, not booksellers/distributors.)

Please photocopy this form for your personal use.
www.HaworthPress.com

BOF04